The
Optimal
Dose

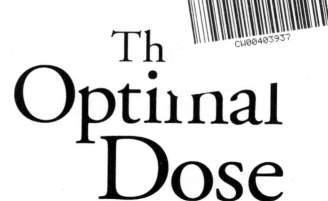

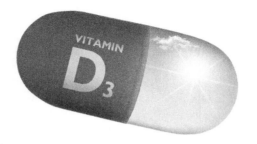

Restore Your Health With the Power of Vitamin D3

Judson Somerville, MD

Author: Judson Somerville, MD
Editor: Nancy Pile
© 2018 by Judson Somerville, MD

Disclaimer: This book is not intended to substitute for the counsel of a qualified health professional or to diagnosis or treat any disease. The reader takes full responsibility for any action taken after reading this material. Improper use of vitamin D can lead to hypercalcemia and in rare cases permanent damage and possibly death. Some individuals due to preexisting medical conditions are more prone to these side effects and should only use vitamin D if recommended by their physician. The reader is advised to consult a qualified health professional before making any changes in the amount of vitamin D, magnesium or for that matter any supplements, vitamins or minerals.

ISBN: 978-1-7326550-0-3
Printed in the United States of America

To my mom—you did a great job.
You taught me to turn human waste into fertilizer.

Luck is when preparation meets opportunity.

—Grant Teaff, Baylor University football head coach (1972-92)

Table of Contents

Welcome to Your Ideal Health with Vitamin D3 Optimal Dosing

This book is part of my mission to change people's health and lives for the better. This book explains my discovery of how all of us can elevate our health through optimal dosing of vitamin D3—what thousands of my patients and I consider a *miracle* vitamin. It offers a detailed exploration of the lifesaving effects of optimal dosing of vitamin D3, one of the most unheralded cures available today.

How can vitamin D3 help you? What health issues does vitamin D3 address? Here is just a short list of the ailments that vitamin D3 at optimal dose levels helps:

- Autism spectrum disorder

- Lyme disease

- Influenza

- Cancer

- Multiple sclerosis

- Obesity

- Diabetes

- Sleep apnea

- Chronic fatigue

- Dementia

My Introduction to Vitamin D3

In 2010 I was desperate. My immune system was noticeably weaker, my sleep chronically poor, my weight a hundred pounds too heavy, and my energy and spirit at a low. On top of this, as a hard-working, dedicated physician for sixteen years and counting, I was taking care of thousands of patients. Just as I was worried about my own health, I was deeply concerned about theirs. For me to give them the care and the compassion they needed, I had to figure out what was holding back my own health.

What was going on with me? Something was missing. Something key to the state of my overall health was missing. And I was desperate to find it. That's the reason behind the life-or-death quest that brought me to vitamin D3. To clarify, my life wasn't exactly at risk, but the quality of my life certainly was. I was constantly septic due to chronic low-grade urinary tract infections and wound infections.

I decided to concentrate on my chronic lack of deep restorative sleep (DRS). I figured that if I could restore the quality of my sleep, then I'd be in a stronger position to work on other areas of my health. It was in my research on DRS, that I came upon vitamin D3 and the possibility that most people in today's world are functioning on suboptimal levels of vitamin D3. Because vitamin D3 plays a pivotal role in the body achieving the state needed for deep sleep to happen, a person at suboptimal levels ends up never achieving that deep sleep state—even after a supposedly full eight to ten hours of rest.

When you fail to achieve DRS, you never feel fully rested, rejuvenated, and recharged. Basically, in the morning when it's time to get up, you're exhausted. Notice this isn't talking about length of sleep; it's the depth of sleep that matters.

It was due to this chronically exhausted state that I began my foray into the study of vitamin D3 and its critical and multifaceted roles in the human body.

Rejuvenated and Robust: 8+ Years Later

Eight-plus years later, I'm about one hundred pounds lighter, a regular deep sleeper, with a robust immune system, and on most days my energy and spirits are high.

What happened?

Upon first learning about the connection between vitamin D3 and deep restorative sleep so many years ago, I continued learning more about vitamin D3. I delved into research on the issue, met up with other medical experts and pioneers, and even did my own research. Eventually, I came to understand the connection between vitamin D3 and multiple systems in the human body. Vitamin D3 plays a key role in the immune system, in the mechanisms involved in deep restorative sleep, and metabolic systems (meaning weight-loss and weight-gain related). When vitamin D3 levels in your blood are optimal, your immune system, depth of sleep, and metabolism are primed to function at their greatest potential.

The reverse is also true: when the vitamin D3 levels in your blood are suboptimal, your immune system, depth of sleep, and metabolism deteriorate.

In my studies, I came to learn that like so many of us in today's modern world, my vitamin D3 levels for years, decades even, were suboptimal. That's why no matter how much I was supposedly sleeping, I couldn't achieve deep sleep and feel fully rested. That's why I was obese. That's why my immune system had difficulty fighting off infection. That's why my spirits were low and my energy too. What I'm describing about myself is what so many other people are suffering as well. It's a condition I've dubbed "winter syndrome," and you can expect this book to explain it to you in detail.

After I made these discoveries and connections, I polled my patients and learned of their chronic sleep troubles. I am talking thousands of patients whom I asked a series of detailed questions only to find that like me, they too chronically failed to get deep restorative sleep. Their weight struggles and proneness to viruses were issues I was already familiar with as their physician. Apparently we all were suffering for years from the lack of optimal levels of vitamin D3. We all were suffering from winter syndrome and didn't even know it.

Winter Syndrome and Optimal Dosing

This book traces the journey I took to restore both my patients' health and my own with optimal dosing of vitamin D3. You see, I'm not the only one who has experienced the miracle of optimal dosing of vitamin D3. After I established an optimal blood level of vitamin D3 and became certain of its benefits as well as it being totally safe, I started many of my patients on the same plan. Now, eight years later, I have thousands of patients who attest to the incredibly, seemingly miraculous, turn in their health due to vitamin D3 optimal dosing. Here are some of those patients' comments about their experience taking vitamin D3 at optimal dosing:

Two years ago, Dr. Somerville started me on vitamin D3 supplements at what he called "optimal dosing" amounts. I was game, as I wanted to try anything that might work. Almost immediately, within days, I was sleeping better. I discovered that I was more rested, had more bounce in my step and more energy. I started thinking better. It was like a light bulb in my body went off and told my body, "OK. Everything is fine now."

Within six weeks I started to notice weight loss—but I hadn't changed my eating habits, at least not intentionally. In the first four months I lost twenty-two pounds. And let me say I was not working out at all as I was too busy and didn't have the time. Today, I'm at 187 pounds (that's down from 240), and I feel the best I have felt in my life. Thank you, Dr. Somerville, and vitamin D3!

—Lewis Wagner, Laredo, Texas

My oncologist says I'm a "miracle" because my type of ovarian cancer has a reoccurrence rate of 75% in the first couple of years. It's 2018—that's five years later—and I'm clean! I truly feel vitamin D3 is a part of my clean bill of health, and I tell everyone I know my story and to take vitamin D3 at optimal doses. Dr. Somerville and vitamin D3 saved my life.

—Laci Moffitt, Laredo, Texas

Within two months [of starting vitamin D3 at optimal levels] I was shocked at my progress. I started sleeping through the night, which I hadn't done in five years. The pain in my legs and arms became manageable. Now I am able to get out, make new friends, and be happy again. I am thrilled! Vitamin D3 has changed my life. I still take the optimal dose every morning. I know I would not be here today if it was not for Dr. Somerville.

—Cathy Hoxworth, Laredo, Texas

I recently went in to have a follow-up MRI done on my back, and it showed that the degeneration had slowed down a lot! I have also noticed that my vision has improved, which has surprised everyone. In addition, my skin has improved. I used to get sick with a cold or flu five to six times a year, but now I don't get sick at all. I am getting the same number of hours of sleep, but I'm getting better sleep, more restful and peaceful. Previously I had high cholesterol and now my levels are way down. I have not changed my exercise or my eating habits at all. So, the only thing I can attribute these positive things to is my optimal intake of vitamin D3. I give all the credit to Dr. Somerville and the vitamin D supplements that he recommended. He's given me my normal life back.

—Brent Mainheart, Laredo, Texas

Please note: you can find more detailed descriptions of these patients' experiences taking vitamin D3 in the appendix at the back of this book.

Optimal dosing of vitamin D3 saved my life, restored my health, and has done the same for thousands of others. This is the miracle that this book lays out for you, so that you too can understand how vitamin D3 works in the body, and from there, you may choose to begin taking optimal doses of vitamin D3 as well.

Book Setup

This book is not intended to be a comprehensive reference but more of a guidebook. At the start I provide background on how I came to be interested in vitamins and supplements. I explain the effect these supplements, and in particular vitamin D3, had and continues to have on my own health.

Next, you'll find chapters dedicated to why and how vitamin D3 functions in your body—and how its levels in your blood, whether suboptimal or optimal—affect particular aspects of your health. When vitamin D3 levels in the blood are suboptimal, winter syndrome results, which then sets you up for a variety of difficult health conditions, including obesity, type 2 diabetes, heart disease, and hypertension. I argue that winter syndrome is an epidemic that most of the American population suffers from but doesn't even know it!

You'll learn how optimal dosing of vitamin D3 can reverse winter syndrome, so you can enjoy a more robust immune system, deep sleep, and improvement in the functioning of your metabolic systems, which for many results in weight loss. You'll find extensive coverage of the relationship between vitamin D3 and each of these key areas of your health—your immune system, sleep, and metabolic systems. Not only will you learn about the disruption that suboptimal levels of vitamin D3 wreaks on each of these systems, you'll also be educated on the benefits that result from bringing your vitamin D3 levels up to optimal.

Along this educational journey I supply many examples of my patients who have experienced turnarounds in their health, particularly in regard to specific conditions they were suffering, after they began optimal dosing of vitamin D3. Because optimal dosing of vitamin D3 has positively transformed my life and the lives of so many of my patients, I'm sharing their stories, so you'll encounter further evidence of vitamin D3's healing powers. That way, you might just ask yourself, "Will optimal dosing of vitamin D3 help me? Does it make sense for me to give it a try too?"

With those questions in mind, here's a list of the various benefits that can result from vitamin D3 at optimal dosing levels. Please notice if any pertain to your own health needs. Optimal dosing of vitamin D3 helps to:

- eliminate sleep apnea,
- eliminate restless leg syndrome,
- restore deep restorative sleep,
- allow you to wake up rested and full of energy,
- prevent or eliminate snoring,
- resolve allergies,
- eliminate influenza,
- correct autism spectrum disorder,
- slow or eliminate dementia,
- slow or eliminate Alzheimer's disease,
- prevent Lyme disease and other viral diseases,
- prevent cancer,
- extend the life of someone with cancer,
- fight off TB,
- restore your ideal body weight, which for many involves the loss of massive amounts of weight,
- change your appetite so you are easily satiated and not craving food,
- block unneeded and excess fat absorption (most),
- boost metabolism 20–30%,
- boost muscle strength 30–40%,
- increase fertility,
- boost energy 20–30%,
- slow aging,
- close wounds,
- fight off bacterial infections like MRSA,
- prevent diabetes,
- prevent multiple sclerosis,

- fight off any of the above listed diseases, and
- boost the immune system.

Because vitamin D3 plays a key role in the immune system, sleep system, and metabolic systems, it makes sense that it has such far-reaching effects—which can be incredibly positive if your vitamin D3 levels are optimal.

Overcome the Resistance

Unfortunately, many in the medical community, government, and pharmaceutical industry don't agree with me. For this reason, I have chosen to include in this book more scientific and medical background information and references than you may want to read. However, I feel that it is important you understand how I have come to my conclusions.

My approach is controversial. Today, any ideas that make others uncomfortable are often attacked. This is especially so when profits, money, or control is at risk. I'm offering this book to share valuable information with a tremendous number of people so that even more people—beyond my thousands of patients—can use it to restore their health. I don't expect to reap any profit. This book is certainly not a funnel to get people into some pricey program I'm offering or to buy some expensive vitamin D3 supplements that they must keep taking for the rest of their life. You won't find me doing any of that. I am not selling any product or program. As a matter of fact, by sharing this information about vitamin D3 with my patients, the result has been that thousands of them have optimized their overall health. The result: they visit my office very infrequently, particularly in comparison to before. Even though their improved health could potentially hurt the business-side of my practice, I am not deterred. I am thrilled for them—and I want the same for you and for everyone. After all, the whole reason I'm a doctor is that healing is my calling!

Let me add that while I feel certain that my theories are valid, I am equally certain that many will resist them. However, I also admit that much more research into the role of vitamin D3 and our health is necessary. As you'll find in this book, I appeal to the medical research community to engage in this crucial research. There's so much for us to learn about what vitamin D3—at optimal levels—does and offers, so please put together the rigorous academic studies. It will only shed more and much needed light on this miracle vitamin!

Obviously, a book can't substitute for direct physician-patient interaction. Your goal should be to work with a doctor who can check your vitamin D3 blood levels and watch for potential adverse reactions. This is something I do for all of my patients who are optimal dosing. Let me add that I believe such adverse reactions are exceedingly rare—and it's a topic explored in the book—but still, you should be consulting a doctor. If your doctor isn't open to optimal dosing of vitamin D3, then find a doctor who is and work with them.

Optimal dosing of vitamin D3 saved—and continues to save—my life. It saved—and continues to save—the lives of thousands of my patients. My greatest hope is that you can experience the miracle of optimal dosing of vitamin D3 too. Don't hesitate to contact me with any questions, concerns, or thoughts as you progress on this exciting journey to optimizing your health: www.vitamindblog.com.

Chapter 1

As My Mother Taught Me

I am a doctor, and I have always wanted to make the human condition better. This chapter tells the story of that journey and my coming to find how vitamin D3 helps make that happen. We'll start with my childhood, then my university years, my life-changing bicycle accident while a resident, and my years as a doctor working to help others' ailments, in particular osteoporosis and sleep apnea, as well as my own life-threatening condition. My journey to discovering vitamin D3 actually began with my mother and her esteem of supplements—which is where we begin.

Growing Up with Cod Liver Oil

From my earliest memories my mother was into supplements. She was always stuffing my two brothers and me full of vitamins, minerals, and supplements. Never was our kitchen counter not topped with jars of supplements. There were all the usual suspects: vitamins C and B complex, along with the minerals, such as magnesium and zinc.

Mom's favorite supplement was cod liver oil. Boy, do I have vivid memories of having to swig down spoonfuls of that stuff! Though my brothers and I did our best to avoid that memorable concoction, we somehow could never get out of it.

Now, years later, I am appreciative of her insistence. That cod liver oil has helped my body develop a better cellular foundation. As an adult, after a spine surgery, a young orthopedist resident approached me to let me know that I had "amazing bones." He went on to say they were so good that I could sell them! Yes, that was a curious statement and one that's stuck with me. In reflecting back on my mother's insistence on taking supplements, I'm wondering if those early vitamins, minerals, and cod liver oil could be the reason for my note-worthy bones.

At any rate, my mom introduced me to this mysterious world of substances that were neither medicines nor food. Growing up, I took supplements for granted and never thought much about them, but that would change.

Another early instance that exemplifies my positive relationship with supplements and that shows my inventive nature happened when I was in high school. At that time, I had a job helping to deliver small portable buildings that people used to store lawnmowers and garden tools in. The shop was on the main street in Conroe, Texas, at a long-closed gas station.

In getting acquainted with the space I walked around the building. Outback on a concrete pad I came upon beehives. As you might guess, I hadn't expected to find them there. As the days went on, I soon sought out the beekeeper. That's when I met Joe Bob who soon educated me on caring for an apiary.

In a few weeks I had my own beehives, one that I purchased from him and another I acquired by corralling a wild swarm of bees I happened to come across. I placed both in my backyard at my home. Joe Bob had shown me how to keep from being stung when opening up the top of the wooden hives to inspect the bees and honey frames. Despite his instructions, being a novice, I was stung many times.

At the time, I had thick, curly black hair, and that's what the bees tried to attack. I assume the bees mistook me for a skunk or maybe a bear. After darting at my hair, which they found impenetrable, they would sting me at the nearest open site on my face—around my eyes.

The area around the affected eye would then swell up quite large, which was usually fine—except when I had a date! In high school appearance is everything. A swollen face didn't encourage courtship. Allowing the swelling to go down by itself would take at least a week.

However, with a pending date, I needed a quicker solution.

Looking for such a solution, I remembered my mother's reliance on supplements. So, I went to the kitchen, looked over her cache of treasures, and stumbled over her zinc tablets. I decided to take several. By the next day the swelling reduction was amazing, especially in comparison to other times when I'd let a sting run its course. The next day I again took several zinc tablets. Soon, by taking this dose every day the swelling subsided in a fraction of the usual time.

Since I was a child, I've liked to experiment, this being an example. And this experience with zinc stuck with me. It wasn't until years later, when I was finishing college that I turned my attention again to the saving grace of supplements, vitamins, and minerals.

Supplements Save the Day, Again

Having a lot of spare time in my last semester of college at the University of Texas, I started training for a triathlon. I would swim a mile or two, run five to six miles, or ride my bicycle forty to fifty miles in each training session.

In the beginning of the training, my diet was the usual for me during college. It would consist of a three-day cycle of eating the same things, a diet typical of a thrifty college student. The first night, I would eat chilidogs, the next night, soft tacos with chili, and the final night Chef Boyardee ravioli. Then I repeated this three-day cycle. While I admit this was not very imaginative, it worked for me, and it was quick, easy, and tasted great to me.

Over time with the strenuous exercising, my appetite changed. I no longer felt a hunger to eat meat. So, I changed my diet to very little meat. At the time I did not connect this diet change to what happened next.

I started developing fatigue. I was so fatigued that I did not have the energy to work out. This was not me, as I loved exercising. At first,

I thought I might have been over-training. My body and mind wanted to go, but I couldn't.

Next, I started going through possible causes for the fatigue: emotional, spiritual, or a problem with my workouts? I ruled those out. Then I realized that the one thing that had changed was my appetite and diet. My taste had changed. I was eating more and more prepackaged vegetables and rice meals with less and less meat.

It occurred to me that something was missing in my diet. Vitamin deficiency was one possibility. I had learned in college biochemistry that vitamin deficiencies can cause diseases, such as scurvy and beriberi. No, I did not think I was coming down with one of those diseases.

Because my fatigue appeared metabolic-related, I figured that some key factor was deficient. I figured the most probable deficiency I could be experiencing was a B vitamin deficiency. I started taking a vitamin B complex, and within days my fatigue vanished. Similar to before with zinc, I now saw how the effects of a particular vitamin supplementation were immediate and amazing. This was another important insight as to how the body works and the way it responds to supplements, vitamins, and minerals. Again, a problem solved with mom's influence.

Medical Training: West and East

During medical school I took any opportunity to increase my understanding of human health. At McGovern Medical School we had an annual retreat before our first year. I participated in this program. While with a group of fellow medical students, I met John Ribble, MD, an internist at the medical school who would later become dean.

While with him he mentioned an annual exchange program that McGovern participated in with the Capital Institute of Medicine in Beijing, China. Loving to travel and the thought of going to a distant place, such as China, was super exciting to me as was the thought of learning about Chinese traditional medicine. That night I decided that I was going to participate in the exchange. The odds were not great as each year they only selected ten students out of 240 to go. This exchange program was to take place during the last months of our fourth year of medical school, so I had a while to make it happen—almost four years!

In the ensuing four years I did what I knew it would take. By working hard, I performed well enough in medical school that they selected me to go. The experience in China widened my appreciation for options beyond traditional Western medicine, as I (like all American medical doctors) was trained in. As a college undergraduate I'd majored in chemical engineering and had not learned much medicine. After four years of medical school, I learned some about Western medicine, but little about other forms of medicine.

The experience in China opened my eyes. Exposure to their 5,000-year-old medical system started me realizing that there were other legitimate systems than what I had been exposed to in medical school.

One of the students I met in China explained the difference between Western and Eastern medical practices. As he saw it, Western medicine was gasoline and Chinese traditional medicine was kerosene. Western medicine—like gasoline—was super powerful, and when all else failed, it was needed. Chinese traditional medicine—like kerosene—was slow-burning. Though less powerful, it was better used to prevent disease.

I was now aware that there were other ways of treating disease. I appreciated and respected Chinese medicine as it promoted interceding as early as possible in treatment to get the best results. Prevention was a powerful option.

The Healing Effect of a Caring Physician: A Firsthand Experience

Upon returning from China with a new understanding of medicine, it was time for "the match." The match occurs at the end of medical school when students find out where they are going for residency training. My match: general surgery at the University of Massachusetts Medical Center in Worchester, Massachusetts. That's where I would spend the next five years of my life. Talk about a new experience in a faraway land! Like I said, I like traveling and the personal growth it brings.

Worchester, Massachusetts was very different than any place I had ever lived before. In time I adjusted to all the differences. It was during residency that I switched my training from general surgery to anesthesia. In general surgery it was not unusual to work one hundred or more hours a week. Now in anesthesia I was only working around eighty hours a week. This difference was huge, so huge, in fact, that I almost felt as if I wasn't working!

This switch in training gave me a significant amount of free time. Again I started exercising, something I had not yet had time for as a surgical resident. As when I'd been training for a triathlon years earlier, I started riding my bicycle again. The Worchester area had beautiful scenery that made riding even more enjoyable.

Shortly into my anesthesia residency while on a fifty-mile bike ride, my life changed. I was out with three other anesthesia residents on a ride to Mount Wachusett and back. On the way back, I crashed while coming down the mountain. This resulted in me becoming paraplegic. This occurred on August 5, 1990.

Going from being athletic to wheelchair-bound was a big change, to say the least. In the past I used my physical abilities to solve problems. Now I could not.

About four months after the crash and into my new wheel-chair-bound life, I began developing serious health issues. This was another big change as before I had always taken great pride in never being ill, except for minor things. I'd never had a sports injury or significant medical issue.

After the crash and once I began developing serious health issues, it then became clear to me that there are degrees of illness. Until a person suffers from a real illness or disease, minor stuff like the flu or a GI bug is nothing. I guess that's why it is so easy for those who have not ever been ill or never have suffered from a chronic, debilitating disease to be clueless or judgmental in regard to those enduring significant illness or disease.

At first, my recovery went well, but as mentioned, four months in, I experienced serious health issues. First, I felt very fatigued. One of my many other symptoms was swelling in my thighs. I would also have night sweats that would soak my bed sheets, and I would wake drained and exhausted.

Because I was also an anesthesia resident at this time, I struggled to make it to work. For the first hour of the morning, it took all my energy to overcome nausea and vomiting, another of the symptoms. It was not like me to show up to work late or miss work. If I did, one of my fellow residents had to cover for me, and that did not make me many friends.

Until this time, I'd always been a great sleeper. Now I was suffering from a lack of deep restorative sleep (DRS). After DRS a person awakes refreshed. This was the first time in my life that my DRS was gone for any length of time.

Before the accident and illness, for me, exercising would assure I had DRS. However, at this time I was too ill for exercise. Though in the past I'd appreciated my sleep, once I lost my DRS, that's when I learned how truly valuable it was. At the time, on a day-by-day basis, I felt my energy drain and a distinct inability to function at my previous level.

As I've explained, these medical issues were new to me. I went and saw many doctors, but they could not and never did figure out what was causing this illness. There was no doubt I was suffering from some illness. Dr. Will, my physician at the time, diagnosed me with myositis ossificans. Myositis ossificans is where the muscles and tendons become calcified in the afflicted area. This diagnosis was never confirmed or determined conclusively.

Despite this unclear diagnosis, Dr. Will did not doubt me or give up on trying to help me. This made me, as a doctor, realize something important: even if the patient's disease is not listed or diagnosed, it doesn't mean that it does not exist. Nor because of that, that it cannot cause them pain and suffering.

Though in so many books written by physicians, they stress the importance of empathizing with the patient, in real life most physicians do not. So many doctors out in practice, unfortunately, believe that if they cannot put a name on what a patient describes, then it cannot be real.

My dual experience as both a long-time physician and a long-time patient has given me a unique point of view. I have found many doctors blessed with great personal health believing they have control over their own health. They also believe that they will always have this control. They can or will not empathize with, understand, or believe patients with a disease that is not diagnosed. This was certainly not me and not my point of view.

After my accident I spent the first month in the ICU at the University of Massachusetts Medical School teaching hospital in Worchester, Massachusetts. Then I spent the next three months away from my residency at the West Roxbury Veterans Administration located in Boston, Massachusetts where I was rehabilitating from the bicycle accident. During these four months my three-year-old daughter and eight-month expectant wife lived in Worchester. They were trying to adjust to what had happened too. At the same time, the residency program was working to make changes as I had made it clear that I was going to return to work. The University of Massachusetts medical center was great in making this happen, but I am sure they were quite stressed. No medical doctor in residency training there had ever become paraplegic and returned to work as a resident doctor. At that time, there may not have been any in the country that ever had done it before.

In May 1991, four months later, right after everyone, including me, had adjusted to my new situation, an influential doctor, let's call the person Dr. Trey, wrote a five-pages typed critical review of me. Dr. Trey had a reputation among the other residents and professors at the medical school of being tough on residents. He usually attacked the brightest ones. At the time I did not know this. With this new undiagnosed disease and a doctor viciously attacking me, my future was in jeopardy.

A month later, in June 1991, almost like magic, my own doctor found the solution for my mystery illness! No, he did not find the diagnosis, but he prescribed a medication named diclofenac, a nonsteroidal anti-inflammatory drug (NSAID) used to treat pain and inflammation. This worked great for me as it resolved the night sweats, nausea, and vomiting as well as the fatigue.

Years later trying to find a safer alternative, I tried every other type of NSAID, but none worked. If Dr. Will had not prescribed this exact one, likely I would never have finished my residency.

With Dr. Will's prescription (not a second too soon) I was able to regain my groove, as they say. Had I not, that attacking doctor may have been able to sabotage my residency and life. Thank God, I was then able to finish my anesthesia residency. Not only that but to also , to thrive.

Soon I was not only chief resident but scored in the top two percent of the country on the nationwide in-service exam. With this start, I then went on to be a practicing physician. Most importantly, through the experience of my mystery disease I learned the tremendous healing power of a caring physician. Thank you, Dr. Will!

Another Challenge

With the mystery disease under control with diclofenac time flew by until I was in my early forties, almost a decade after finishing residency. That's when I was bitten by what I assume was a brown recluse spider, which set off a scary and debilitating downward health spiral lasting ten-plus years.

I found the bite site—on my left hip—upon waking up one morning. Being paraplegic, I had no sensation in this area of my body (though I later realized that I do have intact pain receptors in the tissues in this area of my body). The bite, by the time I saw it, was silver-dollar-sized, pale, translucent, and flat with a black center point.

This bite occurred on the day I was returning home from Big Bend National Park. Once at home, I sought medical care from Dr. Stan, a friend who is a plastic surgeon that treats wounds.

Despite his care, it became worse. For one thing, I'm a paraplegic and I sit for long periods of time. Also, the swelling I had to my thighs from that undiagnosed mystery disease I first had in medical school had never completely resolved. Additionally my long workdays with a full schedule of patients, over time, encouraged the wound to become infected. Soon I ran high temperatures, and the wound grew in depth. It was not long before I became even more ill. What started as a small leg wound had seriously progressed.

Due at least in part to my continuing to work and my wishful thinking that it would go away, soon the bite area became necrotizing fasciitis, a life-threatening bacterial infection that destroys tissue under the skin. This was the beginning of eight years of severe suffering for me. On the positive side, it's what also led me to realizing a life-saving supplement that would end up benefiting not only me but many others as well (and the subject of this book! But let me continue telling you the story of my journey to vitamin D3).

The infection worsened to the point that I was flown by an ambulance-equipped plane to Methodist Hospital in Houston. There they took great care of me. I recovered, but it was long and tough. It took many surgical debridement sessions. That is where they cut out dead tissue. The resulting incision was large. It ran along the outside of the thigh from my left knee to my sacrum. This left me with a large physical void in that region. With large quantities of both IV antibiotics and TLC to treat me, I finally went home.

The wound from the spider bite and debridement remained open and seeping. Due to its depth, length, and bacterial colonization, closing the wound that extended from my knee to my sacrum was impossible. The wound was open, draining, and chronic. To encourage the wound to heal so that it could then be closed, the plastic surgeon from Methodist sent me home with a VAC (vacuum-assisted closure). The suction was supposed to speed the wound's healing and drain any leaking fluids to prevent a mess. My VAC consisted of a bandage connected to suction delivered by a small purse-sized device.

Due to the wound's size and complexity, it required a nurse to dress it daily. A black spongy material placed in the wound kept it open and prevented it from collapsing, thus allowing suctioning to occur. The nurse had to cut the black spongy material so that it fit and filled the wound. The nurse also had to cut sheets of clear adhesive tape to cover the wound and also connect plastic tubing at one end to that adhesive tape covering the wound. At the other end the nurse connected the suction device and a disposable canister to collect the fluids. It took an hour of shaping and cutting the materials to dress the wound. This dressing needed changing every other day. The plastic canisters that would fill with the wound's drainage needed changing once a day. I ended up requiring this care for the next ten-plus years. Let's just say— the VAC plan did not work as planned.

Even with this open wound and the treatment it required, I made efforts to regain my life. I was exhausted, but I had responsibilities: my family, bills, and medical practice. Every day for the next several years I ran fevers and was very fatigued. This chronic illness caused in me anemia and a serious loss of appetite. Even still, I had to continue working and trying my best to live.

At a later point on a visit to the hospital in Houston, my doctor decided to change the type of wound sponge. I'd no longer use the black one. Instead, I would use a white firm one. This change ended up causing a major problem that none of us anticipated until it was too late. The white sponge ended up obstructing the profundus femoris artery to my left femoral head. This caused the bone there to develop avascular necrosis, which is death of bone tissue due to lack of blood supply. As my femur bone joint died, weeks later the wound from the spider bite was spitting out bony pieces.

The result: my femur detached from my pelvis. So when I sat, the loss of support from my leg to my pelvis caused my pelvis to rotate. My body ended up rotating to the left (my right femur-to-pelvis connection was not affected and is normal). This rotation to the left resulted in increased pressure to my left buttock and skin. Now let me explain why this ended up being a major problem.

Imagine a car with low air pressure in the tires on one side. In that situation the lower pressure on one side causes the car's weight to tip to that side. As a result, on the low-pressure side, the tires wear out faster. The loss of my left femoral head did the same thing. This increased pressure while sitting made me at risk for a pressure sore. Being paraplegic, when I'm not in bed, which is most of the time, I sit and put weight on my buttocks. With a spinal cord injury, pressure sores are common and difficult complications. They can lead to chronic infections, cellulitis, bone and joint infections, and even cancer and sepsis.

Years earlier after I got the spinal cord injury, I learned to be very vigilant to avoid pressure sores. To avoid them when sitting in my wheelchair, I used a JAY seat cushion. This special cushion distributes my weight to help prevent pressure sores. Without it my prolonged sitting would cause my skin and tissue to die from lack of blood flow. With the JAY seat cushion I hadn't had to worry about pressure sores. In the previous dozen or so years, I never had even one.

To address this pressure sore complication my doctor readmitted me to Methodist Hospital for two surgeries. One, the femur girdle stone operation, was to repair my dead, jagged, fractured femur. The surgeon would grind down the head of the femur to prevent further damage to the muscles of that hip. However, the surgery wouldn't reconnect the femoral head to the pelvis. Nor would it reduce the increased sitting pressure on my left buttock.

The second surgery was to close the wound. In this one the surgeon would swing part of my left quadriceps muscle to fill the wound. The muscle would supply an extra blood source to the tissue in the wound to close it.

The wound closure and girdle stone surgeries succeeded. Things were peachy after that. I was able to continue to work, support my family, and survive, but not thrive.

Then about three months later, I developed a new pressure sore to my left ischial area, which is in the hip and buttocks area. After only three months being wound-free, again I was suffering with a chronic wound.

You would think that I would realize I had a new wound before it progressed. But being insensate there and having very little experience with pressure sores, I did not realize I had a new wound. So, I began more wound treatment. Over the next seven years this pressure sore required continued VAC treatments, the same as described earlier with every-other-day dressing changes. I continued with constant fevers, fatigue, anemia, and low blood-protein levels. A side effect of constant chronic severe illness was that it killed my appetite. This loss of appetite, thus malnutrition, plus protein drainage from the wound made healing more difficult.

I had a family I needed to provide for, a wife and two daughters. Otherwise, what was the point of all the sacrifices we'd all made, so I could become a physician? I realized I needed to work. My daughters wanted to go to college, which my wife and I were all for, but colleges, especially good ones, are expensive.

I continued working, spending some time with friends and family, but not much else. The strain of my illness was great. This illness and working more than fulltime were killing me. My condition was so bad that it was causing me frequent readmissions to the hospital. Most often this was for blood transfusions or to treat infections. Several other attempts at wound closure failed due to malnourishment.

I worked long hours all week. On the weekends I spent most of my time sleeping to recover from the week's work. My typical workweek routine was twelve-plus-hour days at the office. After each workday I would come home, eat, spend some time with the family, and go to bed early. The problem was my sleep quality.

The sleep length I did receive was adequate to excessive, but despite this was by no means restorative. The thought may cross your mind, "Oh, he's depressed, and that's why he did not get deep restorative sleep." Though I had every reason to be so, I was not depressed as I have always been able to garner satisfaction from a little. As my grandfather, George H. Bowman, Jr., once told me, "If you're not satisfied with a little, you will never be satisfied with a lot." That made a big impact on me, and since then, I tried to live by that.

I strived to make the most of what I had. But as the years wore on, I realized that I was not getting younger, nor was my health improving. I came to the realization that if my health didn't improve soon, I had at most six years to live.

A Lacking, But What?

I knew something was missing. Somehow, I wasn't acquiring what I needed. Like when I was finishing college and training for triathlons, my mind and body wanted to continue but something was missing. In that case, it had been B complex vitamins.

With my illness, other than work, I was homebound. I wasn't able to exercise or get out of doors like I had when I was younger. Exercising had assured deep restorative sleep (DRS) and also helped to relieve stress. I also had chronic pain, which could detract from DRS.

These facts I knew: I had my chronic pain under control, but something was missing, which was consistently causing me to fail to achieve deep restorative sleep. The lack of exercise was a catch-22: by not exercising I didn't achieve DRS to resolve my poor sleep nor strengthen my cardiovascular system to heal my wounds and thus resolve my anemia, so I could exercise. That was not going to change soon.

Stuck with no known solutions, I started examining what I knew. I was more fatigued than before. Often, I was waking several times at night. Even if I slept through the night, I awakened feeling exhausted as though I hadn't slept.

As I tried to figure this out, my pressure wounds became larger. This was indirectly due to my lack of DRS, and its effects on my general health were concerning. My symptoms of fatigue and a weakened immune system worsened. This chronic illness continued to suppress my appetite, resulting in inadequate nutrition. This was further worsening my health. My concerns were increasing, especially because I was aging and approaching fifty.

It was clear my body's immune system and ability to heal were not improving with age. Instead of depressing me, it motivated me to find a solution. It was at this point when things looked the bleakest that I rallied. Here I was: paraplegic, with draining wounds and chronic fatigue. What miracle did I expect to extract me from this?

I went back to what my mother taught me: maybe the solution would again be vitamins, minerals, or supplements.

As I had read an article about the potential positive effects of vitamin D3 and since nothing else was working, I started to experiment with vitamin D3 as a last resort.

Something had to change.

Chapter Recap

Since childhood and initially at my mother's behest, I've seen the benefit that supplements can provide—and as you know from the subject of this book, it is a supplement that would eventually make a life-changing difference in my life (as well as the lives of my many patients and I'm hoping in my readers' lives too).

After the bicycle accident that left me wheelchair-bound, my health became fragile. It was at that time, when I was in my residency training to become a doctor and also seeing a doctor of my own to address my health concerns that I experienced firsthand the difference a truly compassionate and supportive physician makes in the life and recovery of a patient. I've aimed to bring that same caring spirit into my practice as a healthcare provider. It was in this spirit when I noticed my own health deteriorating due to a lack of deep restorative sleep (DRS)—in particular, my immune system being too weak to heal sores and infections—that I investigated my patients' sleep quality as well. I discovered that most of my patients also suffered similarly. Both my own health and theirs was suffering greatly due to this lack of DRS, and something had to change.

Next Up

The next chapter reveals the change I happened upon, which brings us back to what my mother instilled in me in my childhood: the healing power of taking your vitamins!

Chapter 2

Vitamin D3 Awakening

Around this time, I also started checking some of my patients' levels of vitamin D3 and treating those deficient in it. To check a person's D3 level and determine adequacy or deficiency, first we needed a baseline. Table 1, below, gives the blood level values for vitamin D3 from the United States Institute of Medicine (IOM).[1] These guidelines are also the most often used by physicians in the US. These guidelines use the following five levels to determine vitamin D blood levels and degree of deficiency:

Table 1: Blood Levels of Vitamin D and Relevance

Severe deficiency	0–10 ng/ml
Moderate deficiency	11–20 ng/ml
Mild deficiency	21–30 ng/ml
Normal range	30–100 ng/ml
Excessive	>100 ng/ml

The IOM guidelines cite vitamin D3 levels above 100 ng/ml as potentially toxic.

Over the next year I found that my patients were almost all deficient or close to it. This amazed and shocked me. I wasn't expecting to find this. I expected to find the rare person deficient in vitamin D3, but I found deficiencies in almost everyone.

This testing happened during the summer of 2010 when I expected to find patients with their vitamin D3 blood levels at their highest after a summer's worth of high sun exposure. After all, sun exposure is the major source of vitamin D production. Laredo, Texas, where we are located, is one of the sunniest places in the country. So, at the sunniest time of year, when vitamin D blood levels should be at their highest, how was it that most of my patients were experiencing vitamin D deficiencies?

Additional important questions: what's the current recommendation for dosing of vitamin D to remedy a deficiency? What's the current recommended dosing to maintain adequate blood levels?

The current US government-recommended daily doses of vitamin D are shown in the following chart.[2] These values will be important in our discussions throughout this book.

Table 2: Recommended Dietary Allowances (RDAs) for Vitamin D

Age	Male	Female	Pregnancy	Lactation
0–12 months*	400 IU (10 mcg)	400 IU (10 mcg)		
1–13 years	600 IU (15 mcg)	600 IU (15 mcg)		
14–18 years	600 IU (15 mcg)	600 IU (15 mcg)	600 IU (15 mcg)	600 IU (15 mcg)
19–50 years	600 IU (15 mcg)	600 IU (15 mcg)	600 IU (15 mcg)	600 IU (15 mcg)
51–70 years	600 IU (15 mcg)	600 IU (15 mcg)		
>70 years	800 IU (20 mcg)	800 IU (20 mcg)		

* Adequate Intake (AI)

†– Assuming lactating woman does not have vitamin D deficiency.

Since I wanted to help the patients under my care who were deficient, I did my homework. I read up on the recommended treatment at the time for vitamin D deficiency based on the IOM's guidelines.

I started prescribing the doses recommended by the American Academy of Family Practice (AAFP) guidelines that were current at that time. In 2010 the recommended dosing for vitamin D3 deficiency was 50,000 IU once a week for eight weeks. Once the person normalized, they were to take 800 to 1,000 IU per day,[3] the dosing still recommended as of publication of this book. The goal was to increase a person's blood level to at least the minimal recommended normal level, a level above 30 ng/ml.

To my knowledge, until October 2013, vitamin D3 was less available or not available in the 50,000 IU dose. The only vitamin D in this dose readily available in my area was vitamin D2.

Studies have shown that vitamin D2 is not as effective as vitamin D3 in humans.[4,5] It also results in more bone fractures. Being a stickler for doing the best, I waited until vitamin D3 came out in doses of 50,000 IU to advise patients. Once that happened, in keeping with the government recommendations, I recommended weekly doses at 50,000 IU to patients who were deficient.

I soon saw how the weekly doses at 50,000 IU resulted in little increase in patients' blood levels of vitamin D. Even for the patients whose blood levels increased above the deficient state, after a few months when I checked their levels again, they were deficient. My conclusion: the current recommended dosing was not enough.

Only with much larger doses would a person's blood level budge. However, once they stopped that larger dosing, they couldn't maintain those adequate blood levels of vitamin D3. Because the body uses vitamin D3, it constantly needs more. If not supplied, the blood level drops. Whether fat-soluble or not, if there isn't enough vitamin D, the blood level drops. I hadn't expected to find this. After all, there is a lot of sunshine in Laredo.

This weekly dose of 50,000 IU, even when divided into seven days, was twenty times more than what was then the recommended daily dose. This disparity was amazing. Because of warnings that vitamin D3 was so dangerous, I expected if I wasn't extremely careful to see side effects by prescribing such an apparently high starting dose. Yet I found very little effect for a substance that was supposed to be so dangerous and toxic at this high concentration. None of this was making sense to me.

In the patients I treated, this high dose of 50,000 IU of vitamin D3 per week caused zero side effects. Something was not adding up. Thus, based on the then current recommended blood levels, dosing, and replenishing, neither I nor my patients who suffered from a vitamin D3 deficiency improved. There was no improvement in our blood levels.

Off the Precipice

While working to understand this, I made a decision about my personal treatment. As I was so ill and had nothing to lose and everything to gain, it was an easy one. I had seen doctors and received medical treatment. It had helped very little. Yes, it kept me alive, but I was not improving or anywhere near thriving. I decided that I could, like other physicians in the past, experiment on myself by assuming the risk. I had to do something. I had read vitamin D3 might help. What I was looking for I did not know for sure.

I was hoping at least to suffer less from my chronic infections, but I was on an adventure and willing to see where it led. I kept returning to my mom's failsafe: supplements, vitamins, and minerals. No amount of antibiotics, surgery, or other modern medical treatment was helping me to improve. Nor was it slowing my steady decline. I felt like I was on a high, steep cliff covered with loose rocks. The rocks were slipping toward the edge and carrying me with them.

Nothing was slowing my progress toward the edge. Somehow, something was prompting me to focus on this vitamin for my personal last chance. Was it my mother's influence in the past, my experiences in China, something I read, God's intervention, or all the above? Whatever it was I started experimenting with vitamin D3.

My goal was not to try and see if I could raise my vitamin D3 blood level but more to see if higher dosing had any clinical effect on me. I did not think I had anything to lose in my condition at the time. And I was eager to find something new to help all my suffering patients. Even so, I didn't expect to see any difference. As I was so ill and tired that I had no life other than work, I was desperate for improvement, and in retrospect I was hoping for a miracle.

My starting point was with the AAFP recommended dosing. The problem was this dosing had minimal effect on my patients' blood levels. I realized that it would take larger doses on a more frequent basis to raise their and my levels. The most common source of vitamin D3, sun exposure, was not helpful. Most people were not willing to spend the needed time in sunshine to make improvements in their vitamin D3 levels. It was not a practical way to increase levels of vitamin D3 because of the skin cancer and skin aging risks it posed.

Using diet was another option but that required a diet heavy in fish, eggs, or mushrooms, all which had issues. The mushrooms contained and were full of vitamin D2, not D3. The other problems were the cost and the calories alone that had to be consumed to get the needed vitamin D3 levels. Both were huge. This left supplementation with over-the-counter vitamin D3. It was the most available, safest, and cheapest means.

Once I figured that out, I started taking 400 IU capsules of vitamin D3, three or four a day. I noticed zero obvious effects, but no side effects either. I then found 5,000 IU capsules of vitamin D3. I started at a dose of one a day. Then some days I would take several.

Though I was not noticing any changes one way or the other, I continued to take multiple 5,000 IU vitamin D3 capsules a day. I was hoping for a miracle to occur.

D3 and DRS: A Link?

While I was exploring vitamin D, I was, as mentioned earlier, also looking into the problem around lack of deep restorative sleep (DRS), both my own as well as my patients' struggles with it.

I still remember one particular day not too many years after I started practicing chronic pain management medicine. On that day one of my staff members, Pilar, mentioned that all our patients were getting fatter. She was my right-hand person, so her observation caught my attention. I had been so focused on treating our patients that I had not noticed.

Many interventional pain management physicians, including myself, were prescribing SSRIs (selective serotonin reuptake inhibitors). SSRIs are a type of antidepressant used to treat some of the symptoms of chronic pain, like poor quality sleep. Most, if not all, chronic pain patients also do not sleep well.

Weight gain is one of the side effects of SSRIs. It causes weight gain to occur after months to years of use. At the time of Pilar's comment, there were few other good options to treat my chronic pain patients' sleep deprivation.

Chronic pain patients are like the rest of the general population, other than they are suffering from chronic pain, of course. In particular, like much of the general population, they live with low vitamin D3 blood levels and have issues with DRS. I had not put the two—low vitamin D3 blood levels and DRS issues—together yet.

While dealing with my own health issues, it became clear how important DRS is to anyone's health and recovery. Also, my years of treating chronic pain patients reinforced this as did the information I was assimilating from research and conferences, combined with my own observations of the patients I cared for. It became obvious that the lack of DRS was the most disabling aspect of chronic pain and that it caused or accelerated many, many other diseases. This lack of DRS results in many problems along with depression, fatigue, and inability for the body to heal itself.

As I became more attuned to this lack of DRS in the patients under my care, the more it became evident and that a lack of DRS was the norm—not the exception. A person has only to watch TV for a short period of time to see that business people, if not our doctors, have figured this out. Over half the commercials on television concern sleep. They are either aids to go to sleep (e.g., Ambien, Lunesta, and Nyquil). Or they are aids to keep you asleep (Sleep Number mattresses, nasal strips, or oral guards). And if that is not enough evidence, then there are the aids to wake you up the next day (five-hour energy, caffeinated energy drinks, or coffee). This is a hodge-podge way of addressing the medical epidemic level of lack of DRS.

As always, I was looking for ways to improve the health and well-being of my patients. Consequently, once I realized how prevalent and debilitating the lack of DRS was among my patients, I began searching for a better option to treat it. I considered nonprescription options, such as herbal remedies, but none was effective. My patients' lack of DRS was not due to their chronic pain. After I started treating them with medications and/or injections to control the pain, it no longer was a contributing factor in their lack of DRS.

In my reading research reports, I became aware of the almost epidemic prevalence of sleep apnea. I had treated it for years, but only when it was very obvious like when a person snored, and typically the louder the snoring, the greater the obstruction to breathing, and when a person spent periods not breathing during sleep. Now I was forced to take a closer look. So, I began asking patients about their frequency experiencing symptoms associated with sleep apnea, including but also beyond snoring and not breathing. These other symptoms include waking up in the morning with a dry mouth, fatigue, and a headache.

Another sleep apnea symptom that occurs at night is awaking out of a deep sleep. Patients often attributed this to a need to urinate. That might be the case, but as I pointed out to them, if they did not urinate many times during the day, why would they at night? More so, if they had no heart issues and swollen legs?

Also, in those with especially bad cases of sleep apnea, they would fall asleep during the day. Often at the worst time, like when speaking to their spouse or when stopped at a red light. These are all indications that they were suffering from lack of DRS, and in particular, sleep apnea.

After I started questioning my patients on the symptoms of sleep apnea, I was amazed that over half had such symptoms. I had realized that sleep was a big issue years ago, but I was now realizing that despite controlling my patients' pain, they were still not sleeping well. So for those with enough symptoms of sleep apnea to warrant, I ordered sleep studies.

Soon, almost daily I was diagnosing multiple patients with sleep apnea, not only new patients but those that had been under my care for some time. I was sending several patients a week for sleep studies to confirm and then start treatment.

I began this section recalling the day my assistant Pilar commented that many of our patients had been gaining too much weight over the years. Because of this, I considered the reason for this sleep apnea epidemic among my patients to be due to America's obesity issues. What I mean is that my many patients with sleep apnea had also become obese, thus their sleep problems, I figured, must stem from their obesity. I could think of no other reason. (Little did I know that vitamin D3 deficiency was responsible both for the current obesity epidemic as well as sleep apnea and the lack of DRS, but more on that in later chapters in the book.)

Those patients with restless leg syndrome (RLS) I treated with medication. It was the accepted treatment for this. At the time I had not realized that sleep apnea and RLS were connected to deficiencies in vitamin D3.

The sleep studies showed that about ninety percent of the patients I sent for studies had sleep apnea, either central or mechanical sleep apnea. Central sleep apnea was a brain issue that resulted in a person not breathing during sleep because of communication signaling problems with the brain. Mechanical sleep apnea, what most of these patients were diagnosed with, is due to airflow obstructions in a person's nose and mouth during sleep.

What followed was not expected: I diagnosed and treated their sleep apnea, yet their lack of DRS persisted. I even continued prescribing antidepressants, which helped but was not enough. I was not addressing the cause—just the symptoms. I seemed to be approaching the cause, but I could not figure it out. What was causing this lack of deep restorative sleep? I was frustrated by how both my patients' and my own health were deteriorating.

It was also at this time that for a couple of months, I had been taking one or two 5,000 IU of vitamin D3 per day with no side effects but also no noticeably positive results. That's when my life changed. What instigated the change? A talk I attended at a medical conference.

The Talk

Stasha A. Gominak, MD, a Harvard-trained neurologist, was giving a talk on vitamin D3 at a medical conference given by the Texas Pain Society. This was an unusual type of presentation for an interventional pain management conference. As there were no concurrent talks going on, I attended Dr. Gominak's talk. With my recent heightened interest in vitamin D3, I wanted to hear what this doctor had to say.

Dr. Gominak's talk lasted less than an hour and covered how vitamin D3 affects many different aspects of a person's health. She spoke of the connection between lack of DRS and low vitamin D3 blood levels. Additionally, she confirmed my suspicion: the government's recommended vitamin D3 dosing was off.

Dr. Gominak's presentation allowed me to understand vitamin D's effect on our appetite and metabolism that can result in obesity; how it controls our body at night and can influence snoring and restless leg syndrome; and also, how it affects our immune system.

Dr. Gominak's recommended dosing was much greater than that recommended by the AAFP or IOM. She recommended 20,000 IU of vitamin D3 per day for six weeks and then a reduction to 10,000 IU per day. Her dosing would raise blood levels up to approximately the 50–60 ng/ml level.

The fact that she was comfortable recommending such a dose gave me confidence that I too could take that dose. So, I immediately upped my dose. Also, I recommended the same dosing to patients under my care.

Very soon after I saw the beneficial effects. The first and soonest to appear for me was improved sleep, which looked to be the solution to my problems helping patients overcome their fatigue. I was sure too that if I were more rested, it would also help me tremendously.

Another benefit: my patients taking this dose began losing weight without dieting.

Additionally, this dosing solved the problem I was seeing before regarding vitamin D3 blood levels. Now my patients' vitamin D3 blood levels were rising and then staying in the normal range.

From there more and more positive effects resulted, positive effects that neither I nor my patients had expected. This book is going to go into detail about how vitamin D3 works in the body—with a focus on vitamin D3 and its connection to the immune system, to deep restorative sleep, and the metabolism and weight loss—the particularities of these positive effects, as well as the dosing I landed on as being optimal (note: it differs from that recommended by Dr. Gominak).

Chapter Recap

Dr. Gominak's talk opened up my and my patients' worlds to the tremendous benefits of vitamin D3 on the body when we consume it at doses higher than the current RDA. These benefits have tremendously improved the quality of our health and our lives. I want everyone to understand vitamin D3 and all it can do, and that's why I've written this book.

Next Up

Before we get ahead of ourselves, first let's establish some basics about vitamin D3—how it works in the body and its place in medical history. We need to start here, so you can understand how it is that the current American government and medical institutions' recommended dietary allowance (RDA) for vitamin D is so incredibly off. In fact, I found no hypercalcemia, the dreaded side effect of too much vitamin D in myself or the thousands of my patients while we were taking the comparatively higher daily dose that I'll be discussing.

Chapter 2 Notes

1. "QuestAssureD™ 25-Hydroxyvitamin D (D2, D3), LC/MS/MS," Quest Diagnostics, accessed September 13, 2018, https://www.questdiagnostics.com/testcenter/TestDetail.action?ntc=92888.

2. Institute of Medicine, *Dietary Reference Intakes for Calcium and Vitamin D* (Washington, DC: The National Academies Press, 2011), 469, https://www.doi.org/10.17226/13050.

3. Ibid.

4. V. Goldschmidt, "The (Huge) Difference between Vitamin D3 and D2 and Why You Should Never Take D2," Save Institute, accessed Sept 13, 2018, https://saveourbones.com/the-huge-difference-between-vitamins-d3-and-d2-and-why-you-should-never-take-d2/.

5. L.A. Houghton and R. Vieth, "The Case against Ergocalciferol (Vitamin D2) as a Vitamin Supplement," *The American Journal of Clinical Nutrition* 84, no. 4 (October 2006): 694–697.

Chapter 3

Some Background on Vitamin D3

The awakening I received from Dr. Gominak's lecture on vitamin D3 was amazing. Her recommendations reassured me that it was safe to take higher doses. It removed my fear around higher dosing. Her lecture resulted in my accelerated progress. It encouraged me: first, to experiment on myself with much larger doses of vitamin D3. Later, with the great results I saw in myself, it led me to treat patients with these larger doses of vitamin D3.

Dr. Gominak's lecture also helped me realize that too many things concerning vitamin D did not make sense. For instance, how did the Institute of Medicine (IOM), part of the USA's National Academy of Sciences, decide upon such a low recommended dietary allowance (RDA) of vitamin D3? For those of us ingesting these higher doses, are we in danger of vitamin D3 toxicity? If so, how great is that danger? How does vitamin D3 toxicity present itself? How likely is it to happen and at what doses? Also, how does vitamin D3 influence other systems in the body? What are these systems, and why haven't they been studied yet?

In order to get a better grasp on possible answers to these questions, first we're going to explore the body's basic use of vitamin D3.

Vitamin D Overview

There are many types of vitamin D, but the two types mainly offered as supplements are vitamin D2 and vitamin D3. I advocate that you opt for vitamin D in the vitamin D3 form. The two main reasons are that several studies found that vitamin D2 is not ideal for the human body and other studies found that we receive greater benefits from vitamin D3 than from vitamin D2.[1,2]

Vitamin D3 appears and functions in the human body in three forms. There are many other forms of vitamin D3, but these are the major ones you should be aware of to understand how it works and relates to the points I explain in this book. There's vitamin D3 in the "cholecalciferol" form, which is made by our skin, found in some foods, and we can take it in supplement form. Besides cholecalciferol, vitamin D3 comes in two other forms. There is the blood form of vitamin D3 called "calcifediol" and the active form, "calcitriol." These three types of vitamin D3 are what we'll discuss from this point forward in the book.

Skin Production of D3

When human skin is exposed to adequate levels of sunlight, in particular UVB rays, it converts 7-dehydrocholesterol to an intermediary form, which over the next twelve hours or so spontaneously gets converted to cholecalciferol, which is vitamin D3. This is where most people get their vitamin D3.

A person's skin color affects their production of vitamin D3. The darker the skin, the less the production of D3 due to the greater levels of melanin in the skin. Melanin is the substance in our skin that gives it its color. Melanin is able to absorb 99.9% of UV radiation.[3] The greater the amount of skin melanin (the darker a person's skin), then higher and longer UVB exposures are needed, compared to those with less melanin in their skin, to produce the same amount of vitamin D3 from sunlight.

Some sources estimate that some people can produce up to 20,000 IU of vitamin D3 in twenty minutes of sun exposure. However, again, this is only true for some people because rates of vitamin D3 production from sun exposure are so variable. Though there are some charts and formulas on the internet that can be used to calculate vitamin D3 production based on sun exposure, there are so many variables, each adding more error, that I don't consider these charts useful.

Diet and Vitamin D3

In addition to getting vitamin D3 from sunlight, we can get it from particular foods. The table below shows food sources of vitamin D3 as well as their corresponding amounts.[4]

Table 3: Sources of Vitamin D

Source	Approximate Vitamin D Content*
Fortified Sources	
Cereal	100 IU per serving
Milk	100 IU per 8 oz
Orange Juice	100 IU per 8 oz
Nonfortified Food Sources	
Breast milk†	20 IU per L
Cod liver oil	400 IU per teaspoon
Egg yolk	20 IU
Mackerel (canned)	250 IU per 3.5 oz
Salmon (canned)	300 to 600 IU per 3.5 oz
Salmon (fresh, farmed)	100 to 250 IU per 3.5 oz
Salmon (fresh, wild)	600 to 1,000 IU per 3.5 oz
Sardines (canned)	300 IU per 3.5 oz
Tuna (canned)	230 IU per 3.6 oz

Prescription Supplements

Vitamin D2 (ergocalciferol)	50,000 IU per capsule
Vitamin D2 (ergocalciferol [Drisdol]) liquid supplements	8,000 IU per mL
1.25-dihydroxy vitamin D (calcitriol [Rocaltrol])	0.25 or 0.5 mcg per capsule
1.25-dihydroxyvitamin D (calcitriol [Calcijex])	1 mcg per mL solution for injection

Over-the-Counter Supplements

Vitamin D3 or cholecalciferol	400, 800, 1,000, 2,000, 5,000, 10,000, or 50,000 IU per tablet

*– Primarily vitamin D3, except egg yolk (D2 or D3)

The current recommended dietary allowance (RDA) of vitamin D3 in general for most age groups is 600 IU (if over 70 years old, it is 800 IU). Let's look at what that looks like if a person acquired this amount solely through food, namely through drinking milk. Most milk in the United States is voluntarily supplemented, with one cup of milk (eight ounces) containing 100 IU of vitamin D.[5] However, whether this is vitamin D3 or D2 is not known as the government does not stipulate one type over the other. Because it is less expensive in its additive form, it is likely milk producers are using vitamin D2.

To get 600 IU of vitamin D, the current RDA for those under 70 years old, solely from drinking milk, you would need to drink six cups of milk a day, every day. Six cups of milk is forty-eight ounces or four-tenths of gallon. That's a lot of milk to have to drink each day to get the RDA of vitamin D. For a child, it would be particularly difficult to drink this much milk and also have room to eat other foods.

I also suggest that getting adequate vitamin D through dairy is typically only an option for people of Western European descent who can digest milk products. Americans not of Western European descent—minorities—and most of the rest of the world population, are lactose intolerant, so they would need to get their vitamin D from another food source. As you can see from the table, after dairy products, the next main food rich in vitamin D is fatty fish, which tends to be expensive. Yes, other foods, like orange juice, are fortified with vitamin D but again they are typically expensive.

Vitamin D3 Supplements and Injections

Another option to get vitamin D3 is through supplements and injections. As given in the table, over-the-counter supplements come in 400 IU, 800 IU, 1,000 IU, or 2,000 IU per tablet doses.

With this overview of vitamin D, you are sufficiently positioned to understand its place in medical history as well as those other questions about vitamin D posed at the start of the chapter.

Vitamin D: Early History and Consequences

At the beginning of the twentieth century, rickets was a painful and common bone disease in children growing up in smog-covered industrial cities where they had too little sun exposure and poor diets. In the 1930s scientists finally discovered a substance that cured rickets.[6] Similar to how it was discovered that the disease scurvy was cured by vitamin C, scientists determined that the substance that cured rickets must also be a vitamin. Their thought was that because the substance, like vitamin C, cured a disease, was required in small amounts, and also could be given via the diet, then it must be a vitamin. Consequently, they named the substance "vitamin D."

While the discovery of vitamin D as a cure to rickets was life-saving and wonderful, assumptions scientists made at the time of the discovery of vitamin D laid the groundwork for decades of troubling misconceptions, some of which persist today.

Consequences of the Vitamin D Misconception

As already explained, scientists determined the substance that cured rickets must be a vitamin because it cured rickets similarly to how the vitamin, vitamin C, cured scurvy. However, the substance named vitamin D is, in fact, not a vitamin. It's a hormone. Let me explain.

A vitamin, by definition, is an organic substance that humans must ingest in small amounts because the human body cannot produce it on its own. Thus, a vitamin must be obtained through the diet. However, uman skin exposed to adequate levels of sunlight is able to produce vitamin D. When our skin is exposed to sunlight, in particular UVB rays, the human body is able to produce vitamin D. So, by this accepted definition, what is called "vitamin D" is not a vitamin at all. Our bodies can make it. In fact, the human body uses vitamin D as a hormone to perform endocrine and autocrine functions.

Once scientists misidentified the substance, classifying it a vitamin, they then proceeded to suggest dosing levels that would be appropriate if, indeed, the substance were a vitamin. Since vitamin D is fat-soluble, it means that the human body accumulates any additional vitamin D that it isn't using inside its tissues. Any extra vitamin D stays in a person's system. Because other fat-soluble vitamins that accumulate in the body prove toxic and dangerous, these early scientists assumed this must be true of vitamin D as well. Therefore, they determined that the lowest dose of vitamin D that would prevent rickets was all any individual should ingest. Thus, this low "safe" dose of vitamin D became the standard. Doses above this standard were assumed to be approaching toxic.

On top of this, these early scientists didn't explore vitamin D's influence in the human body beyond its ability to cure rickets and its connection to blood calcium/phosphate levels. They didn't conduct any research to learn vitamin D's potential influence in other areas, like its influence on chronic fatigue, sleep, metabolism, osteoporosis, the immune system, and beyond.

Why did early scientists come to such hasty and incomplete conclusions about vitamin D? The answer involves timing. These scientists were desperately searching for a cure to a horrible disease. They were under a lot of pressure to find the cure fast. On top of that, the 1930s was a particularly difficult time in history. World War 1 had recently ended, and the world was on the cusp of World War 2. Resources were stretched thin, as well as morale. For these reasons, it makes some sense that these scientists so happily landed on vitamin D as the cure to rickets, made hasty, error-fraught assumptions about it, and didn't pursue further study.

The Trouble with Toxicity

Unfortunately, this isn't the only poor decision-making in the history of vitamin D3. Let's look at how the current standard for vitamin D toxicity was decided. We'll start by returning to this table[7] first given in chapter 2:

Table 1: Blood Levels of Vitamin D and Relevance

Severe deficiency	0–10 ng/ml
Moderate deficiency	11–20 ng/ml
Mild deficiency	21–30 ng/ml
Normal range	30–100 ng/ml
Excessive	>100 ng/ml

According to the table above, if a person's vitamin D blood level is 100 ng/ml or above, they are in danger of poisoning themselves because 100 ng/ml and beyond is considered toxic. How was this toxicity level determined?

To answer this question, let's look at the given explanation of one of the scientists responsible for this decision. In explaining the decision, the scientist gave these words: "Although current data support the viewpoint that the biomarker plasma 25 (OH)D concentrations must rise above 750 nmol/L to produce vitamin D toxicity, the more prudent upper limit of 250 nmol/L might be retained to ensure a wide safety margin."[8] Now, let's take a moment to dissect what exactly this explanation is saying.

The first component from the quotation to understand is the term "biomarker plasma 25(OH)D." I am going to explain this term very simply: in essence, biomarker plasma 25(OH)D is calcifediol, one of the three main forms of vitamin D3 in the human body and the form of vitamin D3 measured to determine the level of vitamin D3 in the blood. Thus, we can read "biomarker plasma 25(OH)D" as meaning "vitamin D3." With that explanation, the quotation can be read as saying: "Although current data finds that [vitamin D3] concentrations must rise above 750 nmol/L for vitamin D toxicity to occur, the more prudent upper limit of 250 nmol/L might be retained to ensure a wide safety margin."

The second aspect of the quotation to note is that the unit of measure—nmol/L—differs from the unit of measure given in table 1, which is ng/ml. For us to understand the significance of the quotation, we must understand those concentration levels as they compare to the blood levels given in table 1. So, we must convert nmol/L to ng/ml. Here are those conversions: 750 nmol/l equates to 300 ng/ml; and 250 nmol/l equates to 100 ng/ml.

Now let's revisit that quotation and use these conversion rates: "Although current data finds that [vitamin D3] concentrations must rise above [300 ng/ml] for vitamin D toxicity to occur, the more prudent upper limit of [100 ng/ml] might be retained to ensure a wide safety margin."

Let's do a final visit to the quotation to explore that language around the last part of it. In every-day speak, this last part of the quotation, "… the more prudent upper limit of [100 ng/ml] might be retained to ensure a wide safety margin," translates to, "We think it's safer to make that toxicity level start at [100 ng/ml]. By putting it here, people will have a lot of wiggle room before things could get dangerous."

Now that we've broken down the dense language of this quotation, let's look at the complete translation that we came up with. Colloquially, the reason the scientists set the bar for vitamin D toxicity at 300 ng/ml is because of the following: "Although current data finds that [vitamin D3] concentrations must rise above [300 ng/ml] for vitamin D toxicity to occur, [we think it's safer to make that toxicity level start at [100 ng/ml]. By putting it here, people will have a lot of wiggle room before things could get dangerous]."

To return to the question posed at the start of this chapter: how was this toxicity level—100 ng/ml—determined? Apparently, the scientists responsible for determining that level took the data-supported level for D3 toxicity—300 ng/ml—and arbitrarily cut it down by two-thirds to arrive at the official blood level of D3 toxicity—100 ng/ml. Though they knew 100 ng/ml wasn't actually toxic, or near toxic, they designated it as the threshold to toxicity because they thought they were helping people be safe.

Are we safer and healthier as a result of this arbitrary decision?

Because of this arbitrary decision, researchers and scientists since who have pursued study of vitamin D3 have spent time researching vitamin D3 at doses and blood levels so low that little of benefit did or could come from their research. As a result, their studies have incorrectly confirmed the mistaken belief that vitamin D3 is but a minor hormone whose only useful function is to prevent rickets and aid in calcium balance.

Because of this arbitrary decision there is no vast body of research showing the influence of vitamin D3 on other systems in the body. This is why there's such little official evidence of the relationship between vitamin D3 and the body's many systems.

Because of this arbitrary decision, I hesitated in taking higher doses of vitamin D3, afraid that I would poison myself. It's why I hesitated in recommending higher doses to my patients as well. I based my understanding of vitamin D3 toxicity on a standard that was not even based on evidence, but on someone's arbitrary hoping-to-be-helpful decision.

Not only is this arbitrary standard not helpful, but also it has not made us safer and healthier. I argue that this decision has kept people from achieving the health they deserve. This decision has hurt us.

Hypercalcemia, The Face of Real Toxicity

In brief, those decision-making scientists arbitrarily set the threshold for vitamin D3 toxicity at a level much farther below what the data pointed to as the real threshold for toxicity. They saw this as being helpful and offering a greater level of protection to people. What then does this toxicity that they are protecting us from even look like? How does it work? How lethal is it?

Excessive vitamin D3 leads to excessive calcium in the blood, a condition known as hypercalcemia. If you suffer from hypercalcemia, the symptoms will not let you miss it. Table 4 lists the systems of hypercalcemia. [9]

Table 4: Symptoms of Hypercalcemia

Gastrointestinal Conditions

- Moans
- Constipation
- Nausea
- Decreased appetite
- Abdominal pain
- Peptic ulcer disease

Kidney-related Conditions

- Stones
- Kidney stones
- Flank pain
- Frequent urination

Psychological Conditions

- Confusion
- Dementia
- Memory loss
- Depression

Non-Related Conditions

- Bone aches and pains
- Fractures
- Curving of the spine and loss of height

Another symptom not included in the table is heart rhythm problems.

Because individuals can respond to high doses of vitamin D3 in different ways, the best indicator of an overdose doesn't lie in checking a person's vitamin D blood level, but their calcium blood level, as the main and most important side effect of D3 toxicity is hypercalcemia. To protect patients under my care from toxicity, I have had to be vigilant about checking their blood calcium levels.

In searching the literature for vitamin D3 toxicity I came across only one article documenting hypercalcemia in those intentionally dosed with vitamin D3.[10] This article described a ten-year treatment of patients in the Kashmir Valley who were taking prescribed vitamin D3. The authors of the article describe the doses as extremely high: "The dose of vitamin D ingested ranged from 3.6 million to 210 million units over periods ranging from 1–4 months (median :2 months)."

Let's compare those patients' doses to the dose recommended by the United States Institute of Medicine. A patient from the study's collection of cases taking the minimal amount of vitamin D3 would be receiving 3.6 million IU every four months (we're being conservative here by taking the lowest dose offered over the longest period of time), or 10.8 million IU per year. The US government's RDA is 600 IU per day, which equals 219 thousand IU per year. That's 10.8 million IU compared to 219 thousand IU per year. So, you can see that it would take decades to lifetimes for a person following the United States recommended dietary allowance of vitamin D3 to match the amounts of vitamin D3 the patients on the lowest dose end in this study were ingesting.

Of note: it does not state in this article whether those treated also received vitamin D3 from diet or sunlight, which could add to their total intake.

Considering the deep concern about vitamin D3 toxicity that led to the arbitrary decision to make 100 ng/ml the threshold for toxicity in the United States, it is in our interest to note the reports of incidents of toxicity in this article. Because of the extreme margin of error US scientists cited in deciding the 100 ng/ml toxicity level, I, for one, would have expected (before I know what I do now) that all the patients in this article would have overdosed and many died. Interestingly, that's not what happened.

After subjects underwent vitamin D3 treatment for ten years, there were only ten cases of vitamin D3 overdose, which resulted in hypercalcemia. Of those ten cases, all but one fully recovered. The one who died succumbed to sepsis, not hypercalcemia. It is curious that it took ten years at such extremely high doses for the D3 to accumulate and these overdoses to occur. It is also curious that such few instances of overdose or negative side effects occurred despite these subjects taking cumulatively high doses—doses that seem very, very high when compared to the US RDA of 600 IU for vitamin D3.

It's evident that many more studies of vitamin D3 at high doses are needed to determine the true maximum safe blood level. Even still, the cases from this article give further support that the accepted blood level of 100 ng/ml as the toxic ceiling of vitamin D3 is nowhere near accurate.

There have been other cases where people inadvertently overdosed on vitamin D3 due to scam medicines and industrial accidents. Often in these cases the dose was in the high hundreds of thousands (or higher) of IU and was ingested in a day or multiple times over a short period of time.[11,12,13,14] In these cases the people also developed hypercalcemia. There were also other factors that may have contributed to the hypercalcemia besides the elevated vitamin D blood levels. However, none suffered permanent injury. Often before, but certainly once the hypercalcemia resolved, so did their symptoms. In almost all cases where data was available, their symptoms of hypercalcemia resolved when their blood levels dropped below 400 ng/ml. Yet again, this points to the ceiling of 100 ng/ml as the toxic level of vitamin D3 as being far from accurate.

There was a recent large longitudinal study, basically a study of thousands of people for many years, that suggested higher doses of vitamin D3 resulted in increased strokes and heart attacks. However, it was found that those conducting the study did not take into account the effect of vitamin A. The study participants were Scandinavians, and they consumed large quantities of cod liver oil, which contains a significant quantity of vitamin A. Vitamin A is inflammatory, and it was likely the reason for participants' increase of cardiovascular events, not vitamin D.[15] When we look into the details of studies critical of vitamin D3 at higher blood levels, we discover critical facts were not considered. This, combined with the fact that there have been so few studies of vitamin D3 at the blood levels I have found to be optimal—thus all this critical and enlightening evidence is not available—shows, again, the great need for much more study of vitamin D3.

Chapter Recap

In this chapter we explored vitamin D's backstory. Key parts of this backstory include the following:

- The human body produces vitamin D from sun exposure. The rate of this production varies greatly from individual to individual for a variety of factors including the amount of melanin in a person's skin. Other vitamin D sources, excluding supplements and injections, include dairy products and fatty fish.

- Because it cured rickets, the scientists who discovered vitamin D misidentified it, calling it a "vitamin" when in fact it's a hormone. From this error, other errors resulted, including a lack of further study into its multi-faceted role in the human body and very small dosing recommendations.

- The RDA of vitamin D is 600 IU. The vitamin D blood level officially considered toxic is 100 ng/mol. However, we learned that this ceiling was arbitrarily set in an attempt to make people safe. Most scientists found 300 ng/mol as the level at which toxicity could start.

- The needed body of research exploring vitamin D's crucial role in the human body does not exist because the research that has been done, following the IOM's guidelines, uses doses of vitamin D that are simply too low for anything of importance to be measured. I argue that the very low vitamin D RDA of 600 IU and it's too low ceiling for toxicity have had dire consequences on our health.

- If those people who do ingest extremely high doses of vitamin D—as given in this chapter—happen to poison themselves, most make a full recovery. These extremely high doses are above and beyond greater than the doses that I will be discussing in this book.

Next Up

The next chapter uncovers how vitamin D is supposed to work as a hormone in our body. By learning how it is supposed to work, it's easier to understand how it's gone off-course and the resulting havoc that's wreaked on our health. Don't worry—there is a happy ending. In the next chapter I also unveil the optimal dosing solution that my many patients and I have taken for six-plus years, so you too can enjoy optimal health like us!

CHAPTER 3 NOTES

1. V. Goldschmidt, "The (Huge) Difference between Vitamin D3 and D2 and Why You Should Never Take D2," Save Institute, accessed Sept 13, 2018, https://saveourbones.com/the-huge-difference-between-vitamins-d3-and-d2-and-why-you-should-never-take-d2/.

2. L.A. Houghton and R. Vieth, "The Case against Ergocalciferol (Vitamin D2) as a Vitamin Supplement," *American Journal of Clinical Nutrition* 84, no. 4 (October 2006): 694–697.

3. P. Meredith and J. Riesz, "Radiative Relaxation of Quantum Yields for Synthetic Eumelanin," *Photochemistry and Photobiology* 79, no. 2 (February 2004): 211–216.

4. M.F. Holick, "Vitamin D Deficiency," *New England Journal of Medicine* 357, no. 3 (2007): 266–281.

5. Institute of Medicine, *Dietary Reference Intakes for Calcium and Vitamin D* (Washington, DC: The National Academies Press, 2011), 469, https://www.doi.org/10.17226/13050.

6. J. Fischer and C.R. Ganellin (eds.), *Analogue-based Drug Discovery* (Weinheim: Wiley-VCH Verlag GmbH & Co. KGaA, 2006).

7. "QuestAssureD™ 25-Hydroxyvitamin D (D2, D3), LC/MS/MS," Quest Diagnostics, accessed September 13, 2018, https://www.questdiagnostics.com/testcenter/TestDetail.action?ntc=92888.

8. G. Jones, "Pharmocokinetics of Vitamin D Toxicity," *American Journal of Clinical Nutrition* 88, no. 2 (August 1, 2008) 582S–586S.

9. R. Mathur, "Hypercalcemia (Elevated Calcium Levels)," MedicineNet, accessed September 13, 2018, https://www.medicinenet.com/hypercalcemia/article.htm#hypercalcemia_facts .

10. P.A. Koul et al. "Vitamin D Toxicity in Adults: A Case Series from an Endemic Hypovitaminosis D," *Oman Medical Journal* 26, no. 30 (May 2011): 201–204.

11. C. Kara et al. "Vitamin D Intoxication Due to an Erroneously Manufactured Dietary Supplement in Seven Children," *Pediatrics* 133, no. 1 (January 2014).

12. S. Kaptein et al. "Life-Threatening Complications of Vitamin D Intoxication Due to Over-the counter Supplements," *Clinical Toxicology (Philadelphia, Pa.)* 48, no. 5 (June 2010): 460–462.

13. K. Klontz and D. Acheson, "Correspondence Dietary Supplement-induced Vitamin D Intoxication," *New England Journal of Medicine* 357 (July 19, 2007): 308–309, doi: 10.1056/NEJMc063341.

14. H. Lowe et al. "Vitamin D Toxicity Due to a Commonly Available 'Over the Counter' Remedy from the Dominican Republic," *Journal of Clinical Endocrinology Metabolism* 96, no. 2 (February 2011): 291–295, doi: 10.1210/jc.2010-1999.

15. A.H. Zargar et al. "Vitamin D Status in Healthy Adults in Kashmir Valley of Indian Subcontinent," *Postgraduate Medical Journal* 83, no. 985 (November 2007): 713–716.

Chapter 4

Winter Syndrome: Shadow Epidemic

We established that people can get vitamin D from three sources: sunlight, diet, and supplements. We also established that early American medical authorities discovered vitamin D3 as a vitamin that prevents rickets, balances calcium/phosphate levels in the blood, and strengthens bones and teeth—and that they established this narrow understanding of vitamin D3 that has persisted to this day. We established that American medical authorities, fearful of people overdosing, arbitrarily set a ceiling for vitamin D3 in the blood at a level two-thirds below that which research findings indicated was the true threshold after which poisoning was seen to occur. We established that the RDA for vitamin D3 supplementation recommends that most people take 600 IU though there are numerous accounts of people, myself among them, who take tens of thousands of more IU of it per day and whose blood levels are not near toxic nor do they suffer from hypercalcemia much less have an increase in their blood calcium levels.

At this point, it would be reasonable for some readers not to see a problem. Since we can freely get all the vitamin D we want and need from sunlight and our diets, then it shouldn't matter if American medical authorities set the ceiling for vitamin D3 in the blood way too low and that the RDA for vitamin D is also way too low. After all, people have been getting sufficient vitamin D for millennia—way before supplements and American medical authorities, and even America itself—existed. So, we just continue taking in vitamin D as our ancestors did—through sunlight and diet—and everything will get taken care of—right?

Wrong.

We, the people of the 21st century, are not the people of those times before supplements, American medical authorities, and the existence of America itself. Our behaviors, beliefs, and diets are very different from our ancestors, both ancient and more recent. We, the people of the 21st century, are actually suffering from a quiet epidemic due to vitamin D deficiency—and we don't even know it. That's what this chapter addresses: the current epidemic due to vitamin D deficiency.

Let's start by looking at what's going on with people's vitamin D intake, both before and currently.

Our Ancestors and Vitamin D

To comprehend the current vitamin D epidemic, we have to start in the past when there wasn't an epidemic. Before the Industrial Revolution, in general, people across the world did not suffer from vitamin D deficiencies. Not only were they not deficient, but it can be argued that generally most groups were achieving satisfactory levels of vitamin D. We can examine their general behaviors, beliefs, and diets to confirm this.

Before the Industrial Revolution, people around the world, in general, lived according to the seasons. They spent time outdoors, either daily if they were in the tropics or when the season allowed, if they were in the temperate zones. They did not eat processed foods because there weren't any; instead, their foods were more local and seasonal. For those living near rivers and oceans, generally, this meant those people regularly consumed vitamin D-rich fish. Before the Industrial Revolution people did not view the sun as cancer-inducing, so they did not avoid exposure to it. Also, sunblock and sunscreen weren't available to slather on their skin to help them avoid sun exposure.

The Golden Band: Peoples of the Tropics

We will start by looking at people living in the tropical areas of the world, between the two bands of the Tropic of Cancer and Tropic of Capricorn, an area I've nicknamed the "Golden Band." In the Golden Band there's generally two seasons: rainy season and dry season. All year long, generally, there's a more-than-adequate amount of sunlight available most days. Year-round, people in the Golden Band are exposed to an abundance of UVB, so their bodies, typically, have evolved to expect to intake enough sunlight daily to regularly receive vitamin D3. Actually there's so much sunlight and UVB rays that historically in the Golden Band people's skin had melanin in medium to high levels that protected them from the more-than-adequate sunlight exposure.[1]

Temperate Zones

Historically, people living more distant from the tropics, in the Northern and Southern Hemispheres, where there are four distinct seasons in a year, had bodies that developed differently from people in the Golden Band to compensate for their sun exposure conditions. These people depended on the sunlit months of summer (though some of fall and spring too) to collect the vitamin D that would last them through the "lean" times, meaning the dark winter months. To collect the maximum sunlight that would then be converted to vitamin D and stored (remember, vitamin D is fat-soluble, so the body can accumulate it), historically the people in these geographical regions had skin with very low levels of melanin. This pale skin allowed for maximum sunlight capture. Generally, the activities of these people placed them outdoors in the summer months, which allowed for their skin to collect sunlight. These people did not shun the sun or consider it cancer-inducing.

Unlike the historic people of the tropics, whose bodies generally developed to expect a relatively constant supply of sunlight and vitamin D over the course of a year, historically in temperate zones people's bodies had to create great reserves of vitamin D that would slowly get used up over the course of each winter and early spring, only to begin the collecting and storing and using up cycle again. So, unlike their tropical neighbors, people in the temperate zones experienced noticeable peaks and troughs or extreme variation in their vitamin D levels. This extreme variation resulted, itself, in these people as short-lived moments of vitamin D dosing at its optimum and, at the end of winter and early spring, at its most deficient.

The Inuit

Of course, there are exceptions to my descriptions of how vitamin D worked, generally and historically, in people living in the Golden Band versus the Northern and Southern Hemispheres. For instance, you might be thinking of the Inuit who live in or close to the Arctic Circle. You might wonder, "Why is it the Inuit generally have darker pigmented skin than, say, Scandinavians?"

The answer I propose is due to the Inuits' traditional diet. Let's back up a bit for me to explain. It is theorized the Inuit originated somewhere in the Golden Band, thus they had darker skin due to higher melanin levels. They ended up in the Arctic because they were following the rich and plentiful fish up the coasts. Even after they left the Golden Band and headed way north, because they consumed such vast quantities of vitamin D-rich fish—mostly "muktuk," which is whale skin and blubber—their vitamin D3 levels remained high all year long. Consequently, there was no physiological reason to initiate a genetic influence or change, like a loss of pigmentation. The result: the melanin levels in their skin stayed high because they no longer depended on sunlight to get vitamin D.

Native Americans: The First Causalities of the Epidemic

One historic group for whom lifestyle changes led to a profound decrease in their vitamin D intake, and thus their overall health, are Native Americans, the people indigenous to the USA, in particular. Before they lost their lands and were confined to reservations, the lifestyles of indigenous people in the USA allowed them optimal sun exposure and, for some groups, diets rich in vitamin D. They wore little clothing and spent lots of time outdoors, which allowed them significant sun exposure, thus vitamin D3 intake. The wild-caught fatty fish, like salmon, allowed some groups significant intakes of vitamin D3 via the diet pathway.

Once the indigenous people were forced to radically change their lifestyles, many experienced a steep decline in health. They had to adopt European-style clothing, which covered much of their skin, thus profoundly decreasing their sun exposure and also their D3 intake. They were no longer allowed the vast terrain to be migrant or to spend great lengths of time outdoors as they had done traditionally. They had to live on reservations and were indoors more, which also acutely decreased their sun exposure. Their diets also changed, away from wild-caught game and fish to farm-raised meats, grains, and vegetables.

In total, Native American people experienced an extreme decrease in their customized vitamin D3 intake due to the conditions imposed on them. Poor physical and mental health is not uncommon among large portions of the Native American population to this day. I argue that some of the reason they continue to experience suboptimal health is due to their continued suboptimal intake of vitamin D3. I also argue that while Native Americans were the first to get traumatized by the vitamin D-related epidemic simply because they experienced such a massive and swift decrease in their vitamin D intake, most of the rest of us in America are now suffering from the same disease. Though more slowly than our Native American counterparts, the rest of us in America by now have made such great shifts in our sun exposure and diet that we too are suffering the ill effects of suboptimal intake of vitamin

D3. And like our Native American brethren, many of us have started self-medicating in an attempt to find vitality, happiness, and improved health.

To repeat—I offered a very simplified explanation of the overall Inuit, indigenous, and Native American experience and their more recent health problems. Of course, all people's current health problems aren't solely due to the havoc wreaked by suboptimal intake of vitamin D3. However, I argue that it is certainly a factor and likely a significant factor. Let me continue the argument.

Modern Living and Vitamin D3

Though much less rapidly than what happened to indigenous people in North America, many people today, and in the last one hundred or so years, have changed their behaviors, habits, and beliefs from that of our ancestors, such that currently we are not receiving optimal amounts of vitamin D3 through sunlight exposure or diet. Sure, in general, we are receiving just enough vitamin D to ward off rickets, to maintain the balance in our blood of calcium and phosphate, and—excluding the elderly—to allow for adequate bone and teeth strength. However, we are not receiving optimum levels, as our recent and ancient ancestors did. Consequently, many of us in the developed world are suffering a myriad of ways from this poorly understood deficiency.

Sun avoidance—unlike our ancestors, our behaviors and beliefs today encourage us to minimize our sun exposure, either inadvertently or deliberately. Since the Industrial Revolution, fewer and fewer people in the developed world are living and working in accordance with the seasons. For those in the Northern and Southern Hemispheres, where our ancestors may have spent vast amounts of time every summer working outdoors, today we aren't doing that. If we are lucky, we can make the time to get outdoors for a few hours one day during the weekend or a few afternoons a week. Generally, in the summer months most of us aren't spending the needed time outdoors for the sun exposure to happen that would result in our receiving vast amounts of vitamin D3 that our tissues would store to have on hand for the dark winter months.

However, it isn't just the fact that most of us don't generally let the seasons guide our lives that we aren't receiving the needed levels of vitamin D3 from sun exposure as earlier people did. Unlike those early people, we believe that sun exposure is bad for our health and something to be avoided. We've learned that prolonged sun exposure, particularly for people with pale skin, meaning low levels of melanin, will accelerate skin aging and worse—could result in skin cancer. For this reason, many of us in the developed world, when we are outside, we wisely guard ourselves against the sun with clothing and sunscreen. Sunscreen, particularly sunscreen with very high sun protective factor (SPF), is the norm for many people in the developed world. It is wise to protect our skin from the sun because it's been found to be damaging. However, the result of this wise sun avoidance is that we do not develop adequate blood levels of vitamin D3. What you'll be learning in this book is how unwise and unhealthy vitamin D deficiency is; and how beneficial optimal levels of vitamin D are.

We in the developed world, especially, receive very little vitamin D3 from the sun because our behaviors and beliefs are such that we avoid the sun. While this is smart in some ways, it results in most of us not in-taking optimal levels of vitamin D3 from sun exposure. However, if we offset this by getting needed vitamin D3 from our diets or from supplementation, we can achieve that good health.

Diet—generally, in the world over, in developed and undeveloped countries, more and more processed foods are becoming the norm in people's diets. Foods processed in factories have fewer nutrients than whole foods. However, as pointed out in an earlier chapter, vitamin D3 can be gained from eating fresh and canned fatty fish like salmon and tuna. Also, milk and orange juice are often fortified with vitamin D (though we don't know if it is D2 or D3. It's not required to be specified).

Even as modern habits have encouraged many of us to shun the sun, there hasn't been a parallel and deliberate shift in our eating of vitamin D-rich foods to offset the great decrease in vitamin D3 intake due to sun avoidance. And really, why would there be considering US medical authorities arbitrarily set a very low ceiling for vitamin D3 toxicity and also promote a very low RDA of vitamin D, just enough to ward off rickets but not enough to support optimal health? To repeat, yes, we're generally getting enough vitamin D to meet the US Institute of Medicine's recommended guidelines, but that's not enough to allow us to experience robust health. In fact, what we're experiencing is just the opposite: suboptimal health at epidemic proportions. Why? I propose it's due to our extreme decrease in vitamin D3 intake.

Based on the thousands of patients I see in my medical practice, I surmise that most Americans' exposure to the sun is at a minimum, and we aren't making up for that unattained vitamin D3 by eating more fatty fish or drinking eight or more glasses of fortified milk or orange juice each day. Even if we took in more of these foods and beverages fortified with vitamin D as I mentioned before they are grossly inadequate as the amounts added are based on the RDA, which is grossly inadequate. Instead, we simply aren't getting it. We're getting enough vitamin D to ward off rickets, as mentioned above, and, while we are young at least, to maintain the calcium-phosphate blood balance and strong bones and teeth—which is great—but we aren't getting sufficient levels of it from diet or sun exposure to ward off other serious health concerns that result from vitamin D3 deficiency. Actually, we're in a major health crisis, one that's reached epidemic proportions.

Migration and Its Effects—I want to mention too that migration has affected many people's vitamin D intake as well. As transportation and communication have modernized and become available to more and more people, the levels of human migration today are much higher than in centuries and millennia before. Today many people with darker skin whose genetic origins come from the Golden Band are living in the Northern and Southern Hemispheres, and people with paler skin are living in the Golden Band. People today are able to move around and live in areas of the world with sunlight levels that don't "correspond," so to speak, with the melanin levels of their skin. Biologically, physiologically this can pose a challenge for some.

As a result of migrating to new areas of the world, masses of people can find their skin pigmentation doesn't balance with the sun exposure they're receiving. For someone with dark skin living in a temperate climate, the melanin in their skin is protecting them from UVB exposure during the very season—summer—when their body most needs and wants that exposure in order to make and store a massive quantity of vitamin D3 to get them through the winter. Additionally, like almost everyone else in the developed world, people with darker skin pigmentation are also avoiding the sun. They wisely want to protect their skin from skin cancer and to minimize skin aging due to sun exposure.

Due to this sun avoidance and the simple fact that their levels of melanin guard them from taking in large quantities of UVB, people with darker skin pigmentation living in temperate climates, in particular, are not getting near sufficient levels of vitamin D3 to enjoy optimal health. What I'm proposing: this quiet epidemic may be hitting people with darker pigmented skin particularly hard. It is a fact that people in this group suffer a much higher rate of the diseases resulting from vitamin D deficiency than do those with low skin pigment levels. Heart disease, hypertension, diabetes, and obesity, to name a few, are more common in darker skinned people compared to lighter skinned people—and I argue that it's in large part due to extreme vitamin D deficiencies.

Winter All Seasons

I realize I'm repeating this point a lot, but I am simply trying to be very clear. So, let me start by clarifying that today's vitamin D deficiency epidemic doesn't manifest itself in rampant cases of rickets as happened to so many poor urban children during the Industrial Revolution. As already explained, American medical authorities advocate vitamin D supplementation and food fortification at levels that are very low but generally sufficient enough to ward off rickets. So, generally, cases of rickets continue to be prevented by the small amount of vitamin D most children and expectant mothers are managing to intake.[2] However, our vitamin D levels, generally, are so much below optimal that epidemic numbers of people—in my community, in the US, and I argue around the world—are suffering. Before we go into how the epidemic manifests itself, let's look at how it gets triggered.

As given in chapter 3, vitamin D was incorrectly identified as a vitamin when, in fact, it's a hormone. A hormone refers to a substance that the body produces to regulate itself and to stimulate cells and tissues into action. Our prolonged suboptimal blood levels of vitamin D work as a signal telling the body that it is time to start preparing for hibernation, or at least, decreased food availability. The level of vitamin D3 in the blood acts as a hormonal signaling, controlling when the body goes into winter survival mode and when it doesn't. When the hormone that we call vitamin D is at optimal levels, these survival processes do not kick in. But with our current deficiency state of vitamin D, the body believes it is winter and goes into a winter survival mode.

In winter, to survive an organism either hibernates or eats what it can, when it can, and as much of it as possible. Prior to preparing for the winter, the organism fattens up. Sound familiar? Low vitamin D signals our brain that we need to fatten ourselves up. The problem is that we have plenty of food, but reality and logic don't stand a chance against the body's hormonal signaling.

If we could dismiss the messages hormones send us, then either we would have perished long ago by misreading these internal signs, not fattening up, and starving in winter—or we would not need this book! This prolonged winter survival mode encourages obesity, a decreased metabolism rate, and an increase in fat absorption—all of which are crucial to survive short winter periods with little to no food—but not years on end, an issue covered extensively in chapter 7. The low vitamin D hormone level signals our appetite, making us crave the most caloric foods in order to pack on the weight in fat to survive the (so-called) winter; therefore, we become very heavy very quickly.

This winter-survival signaling, as you already know, has a cost on our health. Think of all the diseases and health conditions that stem from significant weight gain, a decreased metabolism rate, and an increase in fat absorption: obesity, diabetes, hypertension, and coronary artery disease, among others. Low levels of vitamin D3 also throw off our ability to get deep restorative sleep, which hinders our ability to repair our body (more on this in chapter 6). Then with vitamin D3 deficiency our gut flora suffer as does our immune system, directly resulting in a weakened immune system (more on this in chapter 5).

This hormonal signaling came about in our bodies as a tool for humans to survive periods of reduced food, which, for our ancestors, typically happened during winters. While the signaling has always taken a toll on the body, the winter, or period it was activated for, typically was short and intermittent, so it was tolerable. It was the cost to survive and was tolerable because it was brief.

The problem is that we, modern humans, established lifestyle norms—like sun avoidance—that have resulted in our vitamin D3 levels being at suboptimal levels for prolonged periods of time. Consequently, the resulting low level of vitamin D in our bodies has inadvertently removed the hormone that blocks us from going into this hormone-driven winter-survival signaling. The result: epidemic levels of people today are in permanent winter-survival mode.

"Winter syndrome" is the name I'm calling the symptoms that result from the body getting signaled to go into winter-survival mode due to prolonged suboptimal levels of vitamin D in the blood. Therefore, winter syndrome is what I'm calling the epidemic that so many of us today are suffering.

As already mentioned, while there isn't a vast body of research on vitamin D, there does exist a small pool of studies that show the ill effects of suboptimal levels of vitamin D3 in the blood, aka winter syndrome. Eight such studies that you can find in the endnotes associated with this chapter have shown the following symptoms:[3–11]

Table 5: Common Symptoms for Sub-Optimal Levels of Vitamin D3, aka Winter Syndrome

- Increased appetite, especially for high caloric foods
- Slowed metabolism
- Increased fat absorption
- Significant weight gain
- Hungry despite adequate food intake
- Poor quality sleep
- Frequent awakening
- Snoring
- Restless leg syndrome
- Sleep apnea
- Fatigue
- Muscle weakness
- Depressed immune system
- Altered (negatively) gut flora
- Seasonal allergies
- Asthma
- Cancer
- Influenza
- Lyme disease and other previously rare viral diseases
- Multiple sclerosis
- Depression

Each one of these requires a lot of explanation, which I do not have adequate space for in this book. Because of this, I will cover the three main symptom areas—the immune system (chapter 5), sleep (chapter 6), and metabolism and weight-related issues (chapter 7). Another reason for not covering every area is there is a lot of overlap. Also, other great books cover many of these areas as well.

A Summer Day Every Day

Imagine a summer in your life when you spent a full day outside. Maybe you were at the beach. Maybe you were doing extensive yard work. Maybe you were watching your children play in a daylong baseball tournament—or maybe you were the one participating in a daylong athletic tournament. Even if you were drenched in sunscreen or wearing protective clothing, you likely got a big boost of vitamin D3 that day outside in the sun, especially compared to your normal intake of it and normal level of vitamin D3 in your blood.

During that day outside in the sun, you likely felt very alive and invigorated but then got very tired that night and slept well.

Why did you get so tired and sleep so well? Why is this? I argue it is due to that massive boost of vitamin D3 produced by your prolonged UVB exposure that day. Sure, other factors contributed, like physical activity and heat. If you consumed alcohol or were relaxing, that would factor in too. Even still, after a long day in the sun, a person might produce tens of thousands of IU of vitamin D3. Yes, this is speculation as there is no exact way to take into account all the factors at play in such a scenario, but it is likely the case. The point: even a short-term boost of thousands of IU of vitamin D3 can give those of us enduring winter syndrome a noticeably positive effect. This brings us to the next point: with the ideal daily intake of vitamin D3 supplements, we can rid ourselves of this winter syndrome and position ourselves to enjoy this amazing day-in-the-sun feeling all year long. Let's explore this.

To start, notice that I am using vitamin D3 supplements as the way to remedy winter syndrome. I am not recommending going outside unprotected and undergoing sun exposure. When average life spans were shorter, full-on sun exposure was not as much an issue, but that is no longer the case. We need to protect our skin from the possibility of cancer and other sun-induced maladies, so I do not at all advocate you have excessive or unprotected sun exposure. (However, I don't advocate complete sun avoidance either. Some argue that there are great benefits to vitamin D produced from sun exposure. Even still, tread carefully in this area because skin protection is very important.) What I advocate is what I call "optimal dosing" of vitamin D3 supplements.

When you do optimal dosing of vitamin D3 supplements, you will increase your blood level of vitamin D3 so that it stabilizes at an optimum level for your body to experience what I call "Madison-HannaH effects." Madison-HannaH effects mean that your body is primed to be at its healthiest. It's when your metabolism is in "summer mode." Your sleep is deep and restorative, thus allowing your body to repair itself. Your immune system is maximally effective in differentiating you from viruses, bacteria, and preventing every aspect of it malfunctioning—from allergies to Alzheimer's to cancer. The body under Madison-HannaH effects is in a state opposite to that of winter syndrome.

At optimal dosing, all the symptoms associated with winter syndrome (listed in table 5) withdraw, and Madison-HannaH effects kick in. Those metabolic changes reverse. You are able to sleep better, and your immune system as well as gut flora improve. To be clear, optimal dosing of vitamin D3 will not make you better than you can be, meaning it will not, for instance, heal a broken leg in half the required time. Instead, it positions you to be the best version of yourself that your DNA will allow. With optimal dosing most people have never felt better in their whole adult lives.

Optimal Dosing

As I've pointed out many times and explained thoroughly in chapter 3, vitamin D3 at current dosing and blood levels is adequate to prevent rickets and, perhaps at least while people are young, maintain adequate blood calcium and phosphate levels—but not much more. When I first began supplementing my and my patients' with vitamin D3, we kept to the RDA. The result: from tests of my and my patients' vitamin D3 and calcium blood levels, taking the RDA of vitamin D3 provided little to no effect. The RDA is simply too small to make any difference in moving your body out of winter syndrome and into "summer mode" or Madison-HannaH effects.

With Dr. Gominak's recommendations serving as further validation, I increased the doses to her recommended loading dose of 20,000 IU per day. It was only when patients took 20,000 IU per day that they reported a noticeable positive effect—better sleep and overall better feeling. However, when these patients dropped down to Dr. Gominak's recommended stable dosing of 10,000 IU per day, without exception, they reported returned sleep difficulties and loss of that state of good feeling.

I continued to experiment and soon increased my personal dose to 30,000 IU per day. After a year or so with no ill effects and many notable improvements, I recommended to all the patients under my care that they too take 30,000 IU per day of vitamin D3. All my future patients started at this dose. And it has been working great.

Initially, I was testing patients' blood levels with the aim of maintaining their vitamin D3 blood levels between 80–120 ng/ml. However, over the years, I've come to the conclusion that with optimal vitamin D3 dosing at 30,000 IU per day, the optimal level of vitamin D3 in the blood should be between 100–140 ng/ml. With this conclusion I'm now calling 30,000 IU per day of vitamin D3 the "optimal daily administration," or ODA, of vitamin D3 and 100–140 ng/ml of vitamin D3 in the blood the "clinical optimal blood level," or COBL, of vitamin D3 in the blood. You'll find I use ODA and COBL regularly in the rest of this book.

For the past eight years my patients and I have been taking this ODA of vitamin D3 and maintained COBL as well. Other than two patients who complained of upsetting stomachs upon starting the optimal dosing treatment, there have been no other negative side effects. There hasn't been a single case of hypercalcemia, which shouldn't be surprising, considering in chapter 3 we went into detail about how findings indicate that hypercalcemia does not start until vitamin D3 blood levels reach the 300–450 ng/ml level.

For readers still worried about toxicity, recall that I also discussed how difficult it is to increase a person's vitamin D3 blood level. Thus, it is extremely unlikely that anyone would accidently overdose themselves at the 30,000 IU per day optimal dose I recommend. Of the thousands of patients whom I have recommended this dose to and who have been taking it daily over the years, the highest blood level I ever saw was 250 ng/ml. It turned out this patient had been accidently taking double the recommended dose. Even at this blood level, her calcium levels were normal. Other than that patient, the highest level I encountered was 150 ng/ml, a level 10 ng/ml above the upper threshold of COBL, but one that I found to be safe in me and my patients. I found ingesting the ODA of vitamin D3—30,000 IU per day–we stayed well out of range of vitamin D3 toxicity.

Optimal dosing allowed us to become what we could and should be. It is not like taking anabolic steroids that make you stronger and recover from physical exertion faster but at a huge cost to your health and by causing a huge imbalance in your system. The natural results of optimal dosing are discussed later in the book. You'll find a chapter for each major area optimal dosing affects, namely the immune system, sleep "system," and metabolic systems.

IU and Dosing

As we've spent so much time considering vitamin D3 doses, let's take a moment to consider dosing of supplements, in particular the unit of measure used for their dosing. As you've read thus far in the book and maybe noticed in the supplement section of the pharmacy, vitamin D3 doses are measured in "IU," which stands for "international unit."

Here is a definition of the "international unit":

It is the units used in pharmacology and is based on the biological activity of the substance. The goal of the IU is to be able to compare these, so that different forms or preparations with the same biological effect will contain the same number of IU. To do so, the WHO Expert Committee on Biological Standardization provides a reference preparation of the agent, arbitrarily sets the number of IU contained in that preparation and specifies a biological procedure to compare other preparations of the same agent to the reference preparation. Since the number of IU contained in a new substance is arbitrarily set, there is no equivalence between IU measurements of different biological agents. For instance, one IU of vitamin E cannot be equated with one IU of vitamin A in any way, including mass or efficacy.[11]

When you compare the RDA of vitamin D3, which for most people is 600 IU per day, to the optimal dose or ODA I recommend to my patients, 30,000 IU per day, then my recommendation seems extraordinarily large. What I want to point out here is that this IU scale, which is based on numerical values, can give us an inflated sense of the quantity of vitamin D3 at my higher dose recommendations.

Let's take my ODA of 30,000 IU of vitamin D3. This appears to be a massive dose. If this were ounces of gold, this 30,000 would be 30,000 ounces, which is a huge amount of gold. However, we are not discussing gold or ounces but international units, IU. When converting IU of vitamin D3 into units of measurement we are more familiar with, 30,000 IU is not that great of an amount. In fact, 40,000 IU of vitamin D3 is only one milligram; 30,000 IU is less than the weight of a housefly.

Thus, by consuming 30,000 IU a day a person is, in fact, taking only 750 micrograms. When you look at it this way, you realize how little a dose of 30,000 IU a day is.

That said, please realize doses are relative. For example, cyanide, is not something you want to be consuming, no matter the dose.

Chapter Recap

We learned that vitamin D historically developed in the human body as a hormonal signaling system. Because the body produces vitamin

D3 from sun exposure, when the body's vitamin D3 blood levels are high, that signals the body that it can exist in a "summer mode." In the winter when there is very little sunshine, the body's vitamin D3 blood levels are low to depleted, thus signaling the body to exist in a "winter-survival mode." The human body developed this hormonal signaling system as a way to ensure survival, particularly in the brief winter lean times.

However, in the modern world, generally we don't expose ourselves to the sun very much. We typically no longer spend time outdoors or live according to the seasons as our predecessors did. On top of that, we've learned that sun exposure can damage the skin and could cause cancer, so the relatively little time we are outside, we avoid the sun using protective clothing and sunscreen. For people with darker pigmented skin, the melanin in their skin adds an additional barrier to them taking in UVB rays, which would then be processed to make vitamin D3. For these reasons, many of us today have inadvertently set our internal vitamin D3 hormonal signaling systems to believe we are in winter-survival mode all year long. What does it mean to exist in winter-survival mode all year long? It means our bodies instruct us to eat what we can, when we can, and as much of it as possible. The direct and indirect result of this is a host of undesirable health conditions and diseases. I call this state of suboptimal health "winter syndrome."

The opposite of winter syndrome is an optimal state of health I've dubbed "Madison-HannaH effects." You can reach Madison-HannaH effects by taking ODA of vitamin D3—30,000 IU—in order to bring your vitamin D3 blood level to optimal (COBL)—100–140 ng/ml. For the last six years, my patients and I have moved our bodies from winter syndrome to Madison-HannaH effects by taking ODA. Physically, mentally, and emotionally we've made vast improvements, which you'll learn about in the rest of the book. My whole aim in writing this book is to educate you about the optimal health you too can enjoy by taking ODA of vitamin D3.

Next Up

The next three chapters explore how the primary systems of the body benefit from optimal dosing of vitamin D3—and how they deteriorate when vitamin D levels are not optimal. The three areas include the immune system (chapter 5), sleep "system" (chapter 6), and metabolic systems and weight (chapter 7). So, next up is vitamin D3's direct and indirect effect on your immune system.

CHAPTER 4 NOTES

1. N.G. Jablonski and G. Chaplin, "The Colours of Humanity: The Evolution of Pigmentation in Human Lineage," *Philosophical Transactions of the Royal Society B: Biological Sciences* 372, no. 1724 (2017), doi: 10.1098/rstb.2016.0349.

2. L.A. Greenbaum, "Rickets and Hypervitaminosis D," in *Nelson Textbook of Pediatrics*, 20th ed., (eds.) R.M. Kliegman, B.F. Stanton, J.W. St. Geme, and N.F. Schor (Philadelphia: Elsevier, 2016), 331–340.

3. A.C. Looker et al. "Serum 25-hydroxyvitamin D Status of Adolescence and Adults in Two Seasonal Subpopulations from NHANES III," *Bone* 30, no. 5 (2002): 771–777.

4. M.F. Holick and T.C. Chen, "Vitamin D Deficiency: A Worldwide Problem with Health Consequences," *American Journal of Clinical Nutrition* 87, no. 4 (April 2008): 1080S–1086S, doi: 10.1093/ajcn/87.4.1080S.

5. M. Rahmaniyan and N.H. Bell, "Racial, Geographic, Genetic and Body Habitus Effects on Vitamin D Metabolism," in *Vitamin D,* 2nd ed., (eds.) J.W. Pike, D. Feldman, and F.H. Glorieux (New York: Academic Press, 2005), 789–801.

6. G.E.H. Fuleihan et al. "Hypovitaminosis D in Healthy Schoolchildren," *Pediatrics* 107, no. 4 (April 2001): 53–59.

7. P. Lips et al. "A Global Study of Vitamin D Status and Parathyroid Function in Postmenopausal Women with Osteoporosis: Baseline Data from the Multiple Outcomes of Raloxifene Evaluation Clinical Trial," *Journal of Clinical Endocrinology Metabolism* 86, (2001): 1212–1221.

8. J.J. McGrath et al. "Vitamin D Insufficiency in South-east Queensland," *Medical Journal of Australia* 174, no. 3 (February 2001): 150–151.

9. R.K. Marwaha et al. "Vitamin D and Bone Mineral Density Status of School Children in Northern India," *American Journal of Clinical Nutrition* 82, no. 2 (August 1, 2005): 477–482, https://doi.org/10.1093/ajcn/82.2.477.

10. S.H. Sedrani, "Low 25-Hydroxyvitamin D and Normal Serum Calcium Concentrations in Saudi Arabia: Riyadh Region," *Annals of Nutrition and Metabolism* 28, no. 3 (1984): 181–185, doi: 10.1159/000176801.

11. "International Unit," Wikipedia, last modified May 12, 2018, accessed September 13, 2018, https://www.en.wikipedia.org/wiki/International_unit.

Chapter 5

Optimizing the Immune System's Potential

One of the major components of winter syndrome is its effects on the immune system. For a reason that is not yet clear, it's been found that ODA of vitamin D3 is critical for our immune system to optimally function. This chapter explores the connection between vitamin D3 levels in the blood and the vigor of the immune system as seen through its response to common illnesses, starting with the flu.

In beginning this exploration, let's do a quick review of what we've learned about the human body, sunlight, and vitamin D3. In the Northern and Southern Hemispheres, there are large seasonal variations in sunlight availability, thus large variations in how much vitamin D3 people take in from sunlight season to season. In the summer months there is excessive sunlight available, and in the winter months there is very little available. To smooth out these variations, the body stores the excess vitamin D3 it gets during the summer, so that it can use it during the lean times, which is the winter months. The body also depends on the vitamin D3 levels to drop significantly—even down to zero—in the winter as this is the body's hormonal signal to go into winter survival mode, which we'll cover in chapter 7.

In winter, when the UVB level drops, the body extracts the stored form of vitamin D3 to fulfill its needs. However, with today's practice of sun avoidance all year long, there's been a serious disruption in this cycle of getting excess vitamin D3 in the summer that's then stored and used during winter months. As a result, all year long, our blood levels of vitamin D3 are suboptimal. Hence, most of us are suffering winter syndrome and don't even know it.

Winter syndrome aside, for those who live in the temperate zones, this seasonal variation in D3 blood levels is key to why we typically develop seasonal diseases. Even with winter syndrome in effect (thus, all year long we have suboptimal levels of vitamin D3 in our blood), during the winter, our vitamin D3 levels are at their lowest. Winter is the time of year when people most often get colds and the flu or influenza. What we've found is there's a direct link between the winter being the time of year when our vitamin D3 levels in the blood are at their lowest and the fact it's also flu season.

Before exploring this connection, let's take a moment to look at influenza. Here are the general symptoms for influenza or the flu:

- Raised body temperature
- Runny nose
- Nasal Congestion
- Coughing
- Muscle pain
- Sore throat
- Fatigue
- Pneumonia
- Death

There are different flu strains that can infect humans. Every year several different strains circulate throughout the world. Often, they are never the same strains, as they mutate creating new ones. Thus, every year our immune systems are challenged with new strains.

There is influenza type A, which is the milder strain, and influenza type B, the more aggressive and deadly strain. Also, there is an influenza type C. These strains can cause what are called pandemics. Influenza, whether type A, B, or C, is deadlier in those with weak immune systems.[1] Those most likely to become infected and suffer the worst effects are the very young or the very old. The very young are vulnerable because they have not had previous exposure or developed any resistance to the influenza strains. The very old because they often have decreased immune systems. Anyone of any age with a compromised immune system is vulnerable to influenza. Those infected have effects along the spectrum of mild illness to death. Typically, 250 to 500 thousand people die each year from influenza, and 2 to 5 million people are seriously ill.[2]

Let's return to that connection we were discussing a few paragraphs ago. Winter is the peak of the flu or influenza season. So why do we contract the flu in the winter? To reiterate, in both the Northern and Southern Hemispheres, flu season peaks during the period of the lowest possible amount of UVB exposure. But this is also after a period of extended low or no UVB exposure. With no UVB exposure we do not produce vitamin D3. Remember for most people in the world sunlight is their main and often only source of vitamin D. Thus, those who become ill have already used all (if they had any to begin with) of their stored vitamin D3. They will not be and have not been producing any for some time.

Earlier I wrote how most of us do not receive enough vitamin D3 by any route—sunlight, diet, or supplements—which results in winter syndrome. Even those who take the RDA of vitamin D3 in supplement form don't receive enough vitamin D3 because the RDA is not near the amount needed. Between the fact we do not produce enough vitamin D3 and our diets and supplements are lacking in adequate vitamin D3, by winter the majority of us are petri dishes awaiting infection. We are deficient in our main augmenter of our natural defenses, vitamin D3. So, we have minimal resistance to the flu and other infectious agents. This is the reason winter is the peak of influenza season.

It should be noted that in 1965 Robert Edgar Hope-Simpson proposed the connection between vitamin D3 and influenza.[3] Though he recognized this correlation, mainly his findings have been ignored. Think how many lives could have been saved if his findings would have been pursued in further studies. However, I venture to wonder that even if it had been studied more, nothing would have come of it since the highest accepted blood levels of vitamin D3 are incredibly substandard due to the arbitrary decision-making around the established but inaccurate toxic level of vitamin D3 in the blood, as discussed in chapter 2.

While the reason behind the relationship between vitamin D3 blood levels and our immune system capabilities is unclear, what is clear is that there is a relationship. I'll soon share the findings of my own and my patients' experiences with vitamin D3 at COBL during the winter months. First, let's continue exploring this relationship between vitamin D3 and influenza a bit more.

Every year those of us living in the developed world are warned about the upcoming influenza season. This is, of course, during our winter. That's when we're told to get flu shots.

In the Golden Band, or areas of the world between the Tropic of Cancer and Tropic of Capricorn, people do suffer from the flu, but they do not have flu pandemics (except those exposed to prolonged rainy seasons where for long periods of time they receive deficient sunlight to produce vitamin D3). Enough people in the Golden Band have optimal levels of vitamin D3 because of their daily exposure to sunlight that there typically aren't flu pandemics (again, except those who experience a prolonged rainy season) in their regions as we in the Northern and Southern Hemispheres experience each winter. Even still, they experience a peak in the flu during the rainy season. The rainy season is when, in the Golden Band, UVB is reduced and people stay indoors for extended periods of time with reduced vitamin D3 production. In this way, even in the Golden Band, the relationship between vitamin D3 levels in the blood and people's immunity levels can be discerned.

Preventative Measures

If enough people have optimal blood levels of vitamin D3, their immune systems will be robust, and the flu will not spread. This is based on the same theory and proven in reality as flu vaccination or for that matter any vaccination. If there were enough people taking optimal doses of vitamin D3, then even during the winter, we could enjoy summer-like flu and cold conditions, meaning no pandemics. When enough people are doing ODA of vitamin D3, we can prevent the flu in ourselves individually, and we can also prevent pandemics of it.

Perhaps you are thinking that we already have the flu vaccine, which is also a preventative measure. I agree that, yes, flu vaccines are intended for prevention. But due to influenzas' rapid mutation rates, scientists, virologists, and medical physicians can often end up incorrect in their prediction for the composition of a given year's flu vaccine.

Each year scientists, virologists, and medical physicians must predict the strains of influenza that will circulate. Then they must develop the correct predicted proportion of antigens to produce an effective vaccine. Because of this guessing game, the resulting vaccine is often only effective against a few of the many strains of influenza. Another big challenge is convincing enough people to receive the vaccination for it to work in warding off a pandemic. These two challenges are great enough such that the flu vaccine is an unreliable preventative measure against the spread of influenza. For this reason, I propose that the most effective preventative measure is ODA of vitamin D3, a theory that I expect you will agree with once you read the results that my patients and I have experienced for eight years and counting since we first began ODA supplementation.

From Poor to Robust: The Winter Silence

It's been eight years since I first started recommending to my patients that they take optimal doses of vitamin D3. So, my patients and I have been through eight flu seasons, one of which was particularly bad.

Of my patients who currently have taken their vitamin D3 supplements as directed, at ODA, they almost never have the flu. Most of those who became ill were ill only in the first year. This was for two reasons. First, it was during the first year, that patients were still so deficient in vitamin D3 to begin with, it took time for them to develop optimal blood levels. Second, in the first year, initially I was recommending the continued daily dose that Dr. Gominak had advised, which was 10,000 IUs per day and then later 20,000 IUs, before finally I set in on the optimal dose of 30,000 IU per day. Even still, it was only a small number that became ill during this time, and it was a more aggressive influenza strain that we had to contend with at this time as well. Let's look at that aggressive influenza strain in more detail.

In April 2009, a new influenza virus emerged in North America—H1N1—and sparked the first pandemic of the 21st century. This virus was not related to previous circulating seasonal influenza strains but had genetic similarity to H1N1 flu strains in pigs, birds, and humans. As this was a new virus and no one had previous exposure to develop immunity, it hit all age groups. In the United States, the Centers for Disease Control and Prevention (CDC) estimated that from April 2009 to April 2010 there were 61 million cases, 274 thousand hospitalizations, and 12 thousand deaths attributed to the virus. Unlike seasonal influenza, most deaths occurred in those between the ages of eighteen and sixty-four.[4]

It was this flu in 2010 to 2011 that made some of my patients ill. Some of those under my care and following my vitamin D3 recommendations of 10,000 and later 20,000 IU per day did become ill. Of those, a few did contract this more aggressive strain. However, it was only two patients that became seriously ill from H1N1. Both were older, had not been taking the vitamin D3 dose I recommended for long, and did not have great health to begin with. Remember, that while ODA of vitamin D3 boosts sleep and so many other aspects of optimal health, it takes time to restore a person's health, especially if deficient for decades.

So, what happened to those two who contracted the more virulent H1N1 strain? Both patients survived. They attribute surviving to taking the higher doses of vitamin D3. Not only that but day-by-day, they noted an improvement in their health, that is, outside of the flu's effects on them. One was my mother.

Since that year we have not had a bad flu season, which is fortunate. Since then—to this day and counting—none of my patients who are taking ODA of vitamin D3 have contracted the flu.

In fact, once my patients became aware of the relationship between taking ODA of vitamin D3 and not getting the flu, they started keeping track. They started noticing which patients in my waiting area were sick with the flu, the ones with coughing, runny nose, and other symptoms of the flu. Once in the privacy of the consultant room, they would try to get me to admit that the person with flu symptoms in the waiting area was not taking the ODA of vitamin D3. Of course, I would not share patient information, but I appreciated that they recognized that optimal dosing of vitamin D3 worked.

About those sick patients in my waiting room: they were either new patients who were unaware of my vitamin D3 recommendations or the extremely rare patient of mine who was not taking optimal doses as I recommended. Though vitamin D3 can be purchased inexpensively, remember, I practice in one of the most impoverished places in the country, so some of my patients could not afford it. For those, I would prescribe it and often their insurance would pay for it, but not always. In a few cases the patients either refused (once or twice) to take it or despite taking it, usually secondary to bariatric surgery, they could not raise their blood levels to optimal levels or raise their blood levels at all despite the dose.

As a physician, it is part of my job to be around sick people. As I stated above, while I have many patients taking ODA of vitamin D3, this isn't all my patients, particularly new patients. So in the past eight years, I've had frequent exposure to flu-infected patients.

Those patients ill with the flu, typically new patients, would often try to protect me from their flu. They would cover their mouths with their elbows when they sneezed. They would warn me not to shake their hands. My response: I would not oblige them. I saw it as important to show to all patients, particularly new and skeptical ones, just how protective vitamin D3 at optimal dosing and blood levels could be. Also, I was curious if what I was seeing was real. Was this dosing of vitamin D3 really making this huge difference? It seemed too good to be true. Also, my other thought: if it is true, why hadn't anyone else proposed it before?

With patients that were sick from the flu, I would touch their hands and get close to them. Guess what happened? I never contracted the flu in eight years-plus. Not even once. Despite my frequent contacts with patients ill with the flu not once did I become ill. My protection: optimal dosing and optimal blood levels of vitamin D3.

Another phenomena occurred that I consider astounding. I call it the "winter silence." This is when for the winter months, I would often go long periods of time and wouldn't have a single one of my regular patients become ill with the flu. This occurred every year during the peak of the flu season. So the rare time a regular patient showed up with the symptoms of the flu, they stuck out. Whereas in previous years—before I started recommending ODA of vitamin D3—it was routine to have an office full of ill patients, patients who were coughing, sneezing, or blowing their noses.

This winter silence had a significant impact on the patients under my care. Before, many of these patients often required many doctors. But with ODA of vitamin D3, soon they were requiring fewer doctors and doctors' visits in general as they were suffering less. Less and fewer ailments were afflicting them. No, they were not restored to perfect health, but they were better. Those under my care became aware of the stark contrast between my office and those of other doctors. This occurred in my waiting room as they often had to wait long periods of time. They would have more time to notice that in my waiting room, as compared to that of other doctors they were seeing, there weren't any people suffering from flu who were waiting to see me. It was and is amazing.

When you compare what was going on amongst my patients with the normal number of people each flu season who become ill, the difference is significant. Yes, the number varies from year to year, but recently five to twenty percent of the United States' population fell ill with flu. With such a range of people getting sick from the flu each year, it is extraordinary that amongst my patients doing ODA of vitamin D3, no one got the flu. I set up my practice to make sure patients were taken care of in as few office visits as necessary, thus I saw a high number of unique patients over the course of the years. Over a period of approximately six years, I saw around 5,000 unique patients, and most shared my advice with friends and family, who likewise started taking optimal doses of vitamin D3 and kept taking it because it changed their lives for the better. Yes, everyone received the vitamin D talk because I was and am that passionate about it.

So much suffering comes about because of the flu. Recently in the United States, 200 thousand people required hospitalization and 36 thousand died due to the flu.[5] Globally there are 3 to 5 million cases of severe influenza and up to 500 thousand people die as a result.[6] Again, the most severe outcomes occur in people 65 and older, very young children, and those with underlying health conditions. These are, again, the ones who are more often with weakened immune systems or no past exposure.

With not only a growing percentage of the population vitamin D3 deficient but becoming progressively more vitamin D3 deficient over the course of their lifetimes—particularly due to increased sun avoidance—then their immune systems progressively weaken as well. In this way, the numbers of people getting infected by the flu will likely increase as well as the amount of havoc the flu is capable of wreaking on them.

Curious is the fact the flu season is lengthening. I attribute this lengthening flu season to the progressive overall drop in the general population's vitamin D3 blood levels. This lengthening of the flu season gives more evidence that vitamin D3 plays a big factor in the robustness of our immune system.

As my and my patients' eight years-plus taking ODA of vitamin D3 attests, by taking optimal dosing people can reverse this trend of a weakening immune system and greater vulnerability to the flu virus. ODA of vitamin D3 to achieve COBL is the best defense as again it is better to not become ill than have to receive treatment. The key is to maintain optimal blood levels of vitamin D3.

Amongst myself and my patients, I have found these levels also built up other aspects of our health. Though, of course, these results are anecdotal, they are still not insignificant. Because my patients realized this significance themselves through their own improved health, they were much more adherent to taking the recommended dose. And this is despite the general tendency of patients—or at least of patients in my experience—not to follow their doctor's advice. However, when my patients experienced for themselves noticeably improved health, particularly in their bodies' warding off of the flu, they continued to take vitamin D3 as recommended.

Vitamin D3 and the Gut: Another Immune Enhancer

With my curiosity and desire to better understand the body and our health it occurred to me there is likely a connection between the gut and the extent of vitamin D3's effect on our health. It turns out there is a great deal connecting them. In fact, the person who figures it all out will likely win a Nobel Prize.

The alimentary canal is what we call the gut, or in laymen's terms, the digestive tract. It's made up of the parts of the body that intake, digest, and dispose of food, both solids and liquids. It starts at the mouth and ends at the anus. It does not include excreting urine. That is the urinary system.

As it turns out, the gut plays a significant role in protecting us from infectious agents, like bacteria and viruses. It makes sense when you think about it because what we eat and drink is probably loaded with pathogens, meaning bacteria, fungi, and viruses that could and would do us harm without this immune system. Considering human beings have been eating and drinking for quite a while and surviving no worse for the wear, the gut's immune capabilities seem to have developed well.

However, a problem arises when a person's immune system is weaker than it should be; when the pathogens ingested are harmful to us; or when the pathogens are greater in number or strength than the body's ability to fight them off.

At this point, let's bring in vitamin D3. How does it come into play in the gut?

First, because the gut contains a significant amount of our total immune system and our vitamin D3 blood levels reflect the tenacity of our whole immune system, the two are certainly connected.

There's a high percentage of the immune system contained in the gut, particularly the stomach and small and large intestines where we digest and absorb our food. Of great importance to our ability to stay well and fight off infections is the flora that live inside the stomach and small and large intestines. Flora is the fancy word for the organisms that live in the gut. Included among these organisms are bacteria, fungi, and viruses. The composition of these organisms, their numbers, and their health play a vital role in our overall health beyond just breaking down food stuffs into the basic sugars, fats, and proteins. More and more scientific studies are demonstrating this fact.

The gut flora is crucial in helping the body kill off viruses, bacteria, and fungi that would and could harm us. Seventy to eighty percent of our immune system can be found in the alimentary tract. Both the organs themselves and the flora living in them help protect us.

If this flora is not there or is unhealthy, we suffer. So, what keeps it healthy? Yes, you guessed it—vitamin D3. As you should surmise, without optimal levels of vitamin D3 in your blood, what I call COBL, meaning in the range of 100–140 ng/ml, the flora has limited benefit.

When your vitamin D3 is at COBL, it is my belief that your gut is primed to function at its optimum. Recent research has found that the immune system is influenced by vitamin D and VDR (which is the name of the vitamin D receptors in the body): "The anti-inflamation and anti-infection functions for vitamin D are newly identified and highly significant."[7] The researchers in this study go on to report, "Vitamin D/VDR have multiple critical functions in regulating the response to intestinal homeostasis, tight junctions, pathogen invasion, commensal bacterial colonization, antimicrobe peptide secretion, and mucosal defense,"[8] all of which affect the microbiome population. Another study reported that the immune system monitors and influences the gut microbiome.[9] Again this is an area for more study, but based on my and my patients' positive response, it makes sense.

Let's look at what the role of gut flora encompasses. For example, scientists have found that gut flora produce many helpful chemicals. It produces many precursors for neurotransmitters and substances like endorphins and enkephalins (similar to endorphins). As reported in a 2012 study:

> The human gut microbiome impacts human brain health in numerous ways ... Through these varied mechanisms, gut microbes shape the architecture of sleep and stress reactivity of the hypothalamic-pituitary-adrenal axis. They influence memory, mood, and cognition and are clinically and therapeutically relevant to a range of disorders, including alcoholism, chronic fatigue syndrome, fibromyalgia, and restless leg syndrome.[10]

Essentially the gut microbiome, the organisms that live there, determine to a significant degree our mental health based on the chemicals they produce and fail to produce. Until recently, this has not been much appreciated.

No, the gut microbiome doesn't produce all such chemicals that the body needs and uses, but when the gut is healthy, the amounts it makes are significant. The human genome has only 26,000 functioning genes[11] whereas the hundred trillion bacteria, ninety-five percent of which are in the large intestine, contain about 4 million distinct bacterial genes.[12] A study in which the bacteria in the gut of mice was eliminated showed that the vast majority of chemicals circulating in the blood, though often later modified, were dependent on the microbiome for synthesis.[13] As one study reported: "These chemicals had a profound effect on mammalian behavior and neuroendocrine responses."[14] For instance, it is estimated that the gut flora produce ninety-five percent of the serotonin, a key neurotransmitter for happiness and pain control, that we use.[15] Without the flora in the gut producing these helpful chemicals that we depend on, the body would either have to use a great deal more energy to produce them itself, or we would have to make due with lower levels. The deficiency of these substances causes negative impacts on a person's emotional state.

Activities like these performed by the gut save our body wear and tear. Thus, we can use the energy we have in other areas, which slows aging and reduces the chance of disease, disease we otherwise do not need to suffer.

Let's look at an example. A healthy gut will protect us from Clostridium difficile infection, often referred to as C. diff. This is a disease that can cause severe diarrhea with abdominal pain. The infection can become so bad that often no amount of antibiotics helps. This can become chronic.

Often chronic C. diff is the result of taking antibiotics, particularly oral ones. What happens is the antibiotics end up killing off the healthy flora in the digestive tract that would have offered protection. When these beneficial flora are diminished or killed off, the immune system is totally vulnerable to C. diff.

When C. diff becomes chronic, it can be quite debilitating. The more that antibiotics are taken to cure C. diff, the more the gut and body are set up to get it again, thus creating a vicious cycle. When this happens, the solution might be a fecal transplant.

A fecal transplant is a procedure where they place the stool from a healthy person into the ill person. The donor has healthy gut flora; thus, their doctors select their stool to donate. They take some stool from the healthy donor and then insert it into the colon of the person whose gut flora is ill. In this way, the healthy flora migrate from the stool into the gut of the ill person to reestablish healthy gut flora. Consequently, if this transplant works as intended, the ill person's gut is able to fight off the chronic C. diff. If it works, it should return the ill person to health.[16]

The problem with using antibiotics or a fecal transplant to fight off C. diff is that it is treating the symptoms not the cause. The cause is the weakened immune system. To treat the cause would be to strengthen the immune system, which is what vitamin D3 at ODA to establish COBL would do.

Vitamin D3 at optimal doses works directly to boost the body's immune system in the gut. In an indirect way it works to assure the gut flora is the right mix. Again, it is better to prevent a disease than to try to put Humpty Dumpty back together again. Ailments to our system may be and often are the result of a combination of things, in particular an infectious agent, low vitamin D3 levels, and genetics. By establishing COBL through optimal dosing of vitamin D3, you are taking out of the equation one of these three factors.

In medical school they taught us how genetic makeup can make a person prone to a disease typically only if there is an environmental stressor. Because of a stressed environment, an otherwise dormant gene for a disease gets activated. By protecting our bodies, there is much less chance these unwanted genotypes express themselves, which is key.

Sadly, what's happening is the opposite. Over the last several decades, due to suboptimal blood levels of vitamin D3, we are seeing more of these diseases due to genetic predispositions. Stressors are coming along and activating otherwise dormant genes, which allow the disease to happen in the body, diseases like AIDS, MS, and chronic fatigue. I propose that by taking ODA of vitamin D3 we can optimize our immune system, so these undesirable genes don't get activated. We'll go into more detail about how vitamin D3 decreases the potential for the activation of bad genes in the next chapter.

Chapter Recap

This chapter uncovers the deep connection between the vitamin D levels in your blood and the hardiness of your immune system, as seen through the lens of the flu. When your vitamin D3 blood levels are optimal, your immune system is primed to fight off the flu. My patients—numbering in the thousands—and I, all of whom have been taking ODA of vitamin D3 for eight-plus years, stand as testaments to this. Additionally, vitamin D3 influences the health of your gut microbiome, which plays a key role in your mental and physical health. When you are taking optimal doses of vitamin D3, 30,000 IU per day, your vitamin D3 blood level will become optimal, which then positions your immune system and gut flora to work at their optimum, so that like my patients, you'll end up visiting your doctor even less frequently than you do now!

Next Up

Chapter 6 exposes the intrinsic connection between vitamin D and a good night's sleep, as well as all the great mental and physical health benefits that are tied to a good night's sleep.

Chapter 5 Notes

1. "Ten Things You Need to Know about Pandemic Influenza," World Health Organization, October 14, 2005, accessed September 13, 2018, http://web.archive.org/web/20051124014913/http://www.who.int/csr/disease/influenza/pandemic10things/en/.

2. Ibid.

3. J.J. Cannell et al. "Epidemic Influenza and Vitamin D," *Epidemiology and Infection* 134 no. 6 (December 2006): 1129–1140, doi: 10.1017/S0950268806007175.

4. "Ten Things You Need to Know about Pandemic Influenza," World Health Organization.

5. Ibid.

6. Ibid.

7. J. Sun, "Vitamin D and Mucosal Immune Function," *Current Opinion in Gastroenterology* 26, no. 6 (November 2010): 591–595, doi:10.1097/MOG.0b013e32833d4b9f.

8. Ibid.

9. N. Shi et al. "Interaction between the Gut microbiome and Mucosal System," *Military Medical Research* 4 (April 2017): 14, doi: 10.1186/s40779-017-0122-9.

10. L. Gallan, "The Gut Microbiome and the Brain," *Journal of Medicinal Food* 17, no. 12 (December 1, 2014): 1261–1272, doi: 10.1089/jmf.2014.7000.

11. J.C. Venter et al. "The Sequence of the Human Genome," *Science* 291, no. 5507 (February 16, 2001): 1304–1351, doi:10.1126/science.1058040.

12. J. Qin et al. "A Human Gut Microbial Gene Catalogue Established by Metagenomic Sequencing," *Nature* 464, no. 7285 (March 4, 2010): 59–65, doi: 10.1038/nature08821.

13. W.R. Wikoff et al. "Metabolomics Analysis Reveals Large Effects of Gut Microflora on Mammalian Blood Metabolites," *Proceedings of the National Academy of the Sciences of the United States of America* 106, no. 10 (March 10, 2009): 3698–3703, doi: 10.1073/pnas.0812874106.

14. L. Gallan, "The Gut Microbiome and the Brain," *Journal of Medicinal Food* 17, no. 12 (December 1, 2014): 1261–1272, doi: 10.1089/jmf.2014.7000.

15. J.M. Yano et al. "Indigenous Bacteria from the Gut Microbiota Regulate Host Serotonin Biosynthesis," *Cell* 161, no. 2 (April 9, 2015): 264–276.

16. K. Doheny, "Fecal Transplant May Treat Stubborn C. diff," WebMD, October 31, 2011, accessed September, 13, 2018, https://www.webmd.com/digestive-disorders/news/20111028/fecal-transplant-may-treat-stubborn-c-diff#1.

Chapter 6

Vitamin D3 and Consistently Good Sleep

My persistent lack of deep restorative sleep (DRS), as already explained in chapter 1, is what initiated my quest that eventually brought me to vitamin D3 and optimal dosing in the first place. For those many of us suffering winter syndrome, a symptom we suffer is lack of DRS, the consequences of which make our immediate daily lives difficult. Cumulatively, over the course of our lives it puts our health in jeopardy. I even argue that lack of DRS is the most widespread symptom of winter syndrome, the most underappreciated, and also the deadliest, wreaking a slow destruction on our quality of life and health. This is what we'll cover in this chapter dedicated to vitamin D3 and DRS.

Widespread, Underappreciated

Lack of DRS, for me, was particularly disabling prior to optimal dosing. I recall waking up in the morning to start a twelve-hour workday and knowing immediately that I hadn't slept well. For lack of a better term, I'd wake and just feel ugly—meaning off, wrong, more tired than when I'd gone to sleep the night before. Sleeping longer didn't help me feel more rested because although the total hours were longer, I was waking up a lot in the night and never achieving that deep rapid eye movement (REM) level of sleep, something we'll address shortly.

In my frequent travelling, I'd often strike up conversations with people. During this time period, I'd frequently strike up conversations about sleep. It seemed everyone I spoke to suffered from sleep deprivation. With a cursory glance at people I could see the typical symptoms of lack of DRS: dark circles with puffiness under the eyes and blood shot eyes. Then I'd ask a few simple questions: do you wake up at night to urinate? Do you feel tired upon awakening after your nightly sleep?

This brought affirmative answers. Most people had been suffering this way for years. Also, people didn't seem to connect their frequent trips to the toilet in the night with that persistent tired feeling. They also thought the need to urinate multiple times during the night was a normal part of aging. They told me that their friends were experiencing the same thing, so it didn't seem unusual. Some even admitted to me that they were awakening sometimes half a dozen times or more in the night. (Note that I'm not talking about people with cardiac issues or swollen legs.)

To me, people's widespread belief that it's normal to wake up frequently in the night to urinate demonstrates the power of self-deception. Especially and despite the fact as they explained to me, during the day, they might only need to urinate three or four times. Most had not stopped to think about it.

The fact is that the need to urinate multiple times at night is not a normal part of aging. In fact, a person's night urination should be in keeping with their day urination. That's normal.

Because most people accept this misconception as fact, they aren't connecting their chronic tiredness to their frequent waking up in the night, and they aren't seeking a solution. I see this as a dangerous cycle that is affecting much of the general population; thus, it's both underappreciated and widespread. It's insidious because people recognize neither the problem nor the solution.

DRS: Repair, Reset, Replenish, Restore

Let's look at what happens in the body during DRS, so you have a strong understanding of how important it is.

A person's sleep cycles across five stages, with the most deep and healing stage of sleep called the rapid eye movement (REM) stage. REM sleep is crucial, and when we are deprived of it, our memory, our mood, and health are negatively affected. REM sleep is also when intense dreaming occurs. When a person doesn't reach the REM phase of sleep or when their REM phase is interrupted, that's when they suffer a lack of DRS.

Though it is important that the body—the arms, legs, hands, feet, etc.—not move throughout sleep, it is particularly an issue during REM sleep as that is when we dream intensely and our body is energized. The problem with intense dreaming is that the body wants to act out those dreams—it wants to start walking, running, sitting, reaching, or whatever is happening in the dream. This is a problem because if the body moves, it wakes the person who is sleeping. So, the body must ensure that there's no movement during the REM cycle of sleep. And this is where vitamin D3 enters the picture.

The control of muscles' nerves starts in the brain. Studies have shown that vitamin D receptors are found throughout the brain and in areas that control motor function.[1] An important function of vitamin D3 is to interact with the cerebral cortex, the part of the brain that controls skeletal muscle function, particularly in the arms and legs, to prevent their activation during the REM cycle of deep restorative sleep.[2]

To simplify it, then, when you have COBL, meaning your vitamin D3 blood levels are in the range of 100–140 ng/ml, then your brain can activate muscle paralysis during sleep—and this is a good thing. While dreaming in this energized state, if the body is not paralyzed, it will act out these dreams—meaning the arms and legs will move. Consequently, if we thrash about, we would disrupt our sleep cycle and pull ourselves out of sleep, thus never achieving REM sleep and DRS. By paralyzing the skeletal muscles, the body is stabilized for several critical functions to occur while in DRS.

Before looking at those critical functions, I want to note that this muscle paralysis does not affect those muscles under autonomic nerve control, muscles like the heart, intestines, and the central part of the diaphragm.

Let's return to vitamin D3 and skeletal muscle paralysis. When the skeletal muscles are paralyzed, the body is stabilized for critical cleaning and repairing processes to happen, both in the brain and in other parts of the body. Let's start by looking at the brain.

The brain needs to clean itself and repair its cells on a daily basis. When we're in REM sleep and the body is paralyzed, the brain actually contracts 30 to 40 percent. I was actually quite surprised when I learned that during DRS, like during REM sleep, the body allows glymphatic drainage of the brain. That's when the brain contracts in order to drain out water and waste. It's a way of cleaning itself. This system of brain drainage was only recently discovered.

As it takes time to contract the brain to this degree, the brain must be on autopilot. If the skeletal muscles are active, then the brain cannot complete this process.

The glymphatic system functions best with the brain contracted. That's why when you are abruptly woken out of a profound DRS, it can take you a moment to come around. Or you might even be confused about where you are or what the day, time, or season is. That is because the brain is trying to expand back to its normal size.

With optimal blood levels of vitamin D3, muscle impulses get blocked and skeletal muscle body paralysis gets put into effect so that when in REM sleep, the brain goes into a deep stable state. In this state the brain organizes itself, taking account of new information acquired, integrating the new information with what is already known, and editing out unimportant information.

Because it may be of interest to readers who do a lot of travelling, those of us who do optimal vitamin D3 dosing have noticed that our struggle with jet lag has decreased considerably. I attribute this to the effect of optimal dosing of vitamin D3 on the brain's increased ability to adjust to time zones. Again, this is anecdotal, but from my personal experience and those who have used optimal dosing as discussed here, we have found adjusting to new time zones much easier. Now that we are getting DRS, it appears our bodies are able to achieve that paralysis state necessary for the brain and other parts of the body to do the needed repairing and restoring. Hence, the brain is able to restore itself and adjust to the abrupt changes posed by jet lag.

During the REM portion of DRS when the skeletal muscles are paralyzed, this allows continual cleaning and restoration to happen both in the brain and the whole body. When the body is in this stable state, it allows the release of hormones to stimulate cellular repair. Also, stem cells can travel to the site of damaged cells, divide to fill the area of damage, and then start the cell's function again.

The takeaway: when you have optimal blood levels of vitamin D3, then the brain is able to activate the skeletal muscle paralysis, which is required for these imperative cleaning, repairing, and replenishing processes to happen in the brain and all over the body. When you don't have sufficient vitamin D3, you'll suffer a chronic lack of DRS, which results in an array of undesirable scenarios playing out. That's what we'll talk about next.

Suboptimal Vitamin D3, Suboptimal DRS, Suboptimal All Around

When a person has below optimal blood levels of vitamin D3, problems occur around the skeletal muscle paralysis. Without optimal blood levels of vitamin D3, the skeletal muscles, essentially, misbehave. They either become too greatly paralyzed, too little paralyzed, or fluctuate between these two extreme states—all of which are undesirable.

In those who have issues with becoming too greatly paralyzed, it causes the throat muscles to weaken such that they do not keep the throat or airway open. Instead, the throat/airway becomes more obstructed. This results in obstruction of breathing. It progresses to snoring. Depending on many factors, it can result in louder snoring and longer periods of total obstruction. The greater the periods of obstruction, then the greater the decrease in blood oxygen levels and increase in carbon dioxide levels. The result: the brain forces the person to awaken enough to breathe. Over time, this is unhealthy and causes mechanical sleep apnea. This disrupts the person, throwing them out of REM and DRS sleep, which means the body is not repairing itself, organizing or cleaning the brain. A host of negative consequences result because of that.

Suboptimal blood levels of vitamin D3 also cause muscles to be weaker and the person to put on fat. Both these factors affect the throat and breathing during REM sleep.

The opposite effect on breathing during sleep can occur too. That is with less than optimal blood levels of vitamin D3, the cerebral cortex area of the brain can cause the skeletal muscles to become less and less paralyzed during sleep, which is called restless leg syndrome (RLS). In this case, the person will move their body limbs during sleep, such that their sleep may become disrupted and they end up waking themselves. The level of vitamin D3 deficiency seems to affect this, meaning the less the muscles are paralyzed and the greater the muscle movement occurs.

Certainly, this is more of an issue during REM sleep, but it can occur at any time while a person is asleep, as the brain center controlling paralysis is malfunctioning. Even if individuals stay asleep as their body thrashes about, they never achieve the needed DRS or REM stage of sleep, which results in their brain and body not getting needed repairs. Consequently, even after a long night of sleep, the sleeper in this too little paralyzed state, will wake up very tired and groggy.

Whether too great or too little paralysis occurs due to suboptimal levels of vitamin D3 in the blood, a person suffers. On one extreme is sleep apnea and the other is restless leg syndrome. Whether it is too great or too little paralysis, instead of continuous and prolonged deep restorative sleep with regular REM cycles occurring, sleep is disrupted. The degree of wakefulness during these disruptions is often minor. However, the point is the person is not achieving DRS or REM sleep cycles. They wake exhausted. When this becomes the norm over months, years, and decades, this is chronic lack of DRS. The results are chronic deterioration of the body and brain function.

Sleep and Vitamin D3 Studies

Finding research that connects vitamin D3 and sleep is difficult because, as mentioned before, the doses of vitamin D3 used in studies are too low. That said, the effect of vitamin D3 on DRS is so strong that even at doses significantly below optimal, studies reveal this crucial connection. A 2017 study showed a significant improvement in sleep in those taking vitamin D3 versus a placebo.[3] In this study 44 subjects were taking 50,000 IUs of vitamin D3 per two weeks—thus, a dose equivalent of 3,415 IUs per day—and 45 subjects were taking a placebo. The findings: the sleep quality scores of those taking vitamin D3 were significantly greater than those taking the placebo. Though the dose equivalent of 3,415 IUs per day is significantly lower than our ODA of 30,000 IUs, I want to recognize that 3,415 IUs per day is much higher than the US government's recommended 600 IUs per day. In this way, these results support a trend showing higher doses of vitamin D3 are better.

Another study from 2015 showed that in 3,048 older men, those with higher vitamin D levels slept longer than those with lower levels.[4] A 2014 study also found an association with vitamin D and longer sleep.[5] A 2015 study that found correlation between sleep apnea and Asian people (the first study I am aware of that demonstrates this) also demonstrated that vitamin D levels affect sleep, with higher levels resulting in better sleep.[6] These studies indicate that researchers are showing more interest in vitamin D and sleep, but unfortunately these studies continue to test vitamin D3 at very low doses.

Both from these studies and from the chapter's explanation of optimal and suboptimal vitamin D3 levels in the blood and the respective impact on the body's ability to achieve deep restorative sleep, I hope that you are well on your way to being convinced that taking vitamin

D3 at ODA is incredibly important for your health and wellbeing. Let's add to your education about the importance of vitamin D3 by examining the impact of chronic lack of DRS on a person's quality of life and health.

Lack of DRS: Its Impact

I think it is fairly apparent that on a daily basis, the chronic lack of deep restorative sleep will result in a person feeling exhausted, drained, not at a hundred percent. And what about the long term? What is the long-term effect of lack of DRS?

A chronic lack of DRS leads to a slew of health issues. These health issues include hypertension, coronary artery disease, peripheral vascular disease, cancer, obesity, mental health diseases, infectious diseases—and an overall increase in the aging process. It should be noted that these are either a direct result of suboptimal blood levels of vitamin D3 and/or indirect effects of the body's inability to get DRS and heal and clean itself. When the body can't heal and clean itself, it ages more rapidly. Let's look at how that aging happens, and also notice the role vitamin D3 plays.

D3 and Telomeres

We've already learned how suboptimal levels of vitamin D3 contribute to lack of DRS. Now we'll look at how lack of DRS contributes to aging. Interestingly, you'll find that vitamin D3 doesn't only factor into this in its effect on DRS, but also in its effect on the inner workings of cells. Vitamin D3 affects aging—either accelerating or decelerating it—via two avenues, which is all the more reason to make sure you are at COBL, meaning your vitamin D3 blood levels are in the range of 100–140 ng/ml.

Vitamin D3 influences the rate a person ages not only by way of its effect on DRS but also in how vitamin D3 affects the telomeres of cells. For a person to stay alive, the cells in their body must replicate. These replications replace damaged or dead cells, so that all parts of the body can continue functioning optimally. As long as cells, in general, are replicating, a person stays healthy and alive.

Telomeres cap the ends of chromosomes in our body's cells to protect the chromosome from degradation and to stabilize it. To repair damages in a cell or replace "dead" cells, the cell simply divides (or replicates) itself. With each cell replication, telomeres get shorter. Eventually, telomeres get too short to do their job. This is when cells stop dividing (or replicating) to repair damaged or dead cells. These cells can live on, but now to repair damaged areas they cannot produce new cells (via replication) but instead fill the defect with scar tissue. This "fix" is damaging as healthy cells have unique functions, which scar tissue cannot replicate. Think of a muscle full of healthy muscle cells versus one with half the muscle cells replaced with scar tissue. Do you want your heart, a muscle, to be made up of cells or scar tissue? Thus, over time this scar-filled cell (or organ whose cells are replaced with scar tissue) will reduce its proper functioning so that a person loses cells, then organs, and then the entire body fails, accelerating death. Thus, the length of a person's telomeres determines how many cell divisions (i.e., replications, which result in new and undamaged cells) can take place. The longer the telomere, the more cell divisions a cell can undergo. The longer the telomere, the greater its ability to keep the organs, and thus the person, in ideal health. You can think of a telomere as a sort of "aging clock" in a person's cells, with the telomere length representing a person's "biological" age, as opposed to "chronological" age.

Researchers have found that vitamin D3 plays an important role in telomere length and thus cell replication and aging.[7] However, exactly how vitamin D3 plays this role is still unclear and being studied. Some scientists hypothesize that vitamin D3 plays a direct role with telomeres in cell replication in one of two ways (they are still studying to determine which way or whether it is both). One of these ways is that vitamin D3 slows aging by increasing the length of telomeres.

Remember, the longer the physical length of telomeres, the greater the number of divisions a cell can undergo, thus the longer the life of the cell, thus the person.

The other way vitamin D3 may directly affect aging is that it prevents the shortening of telomeres at a certain point in the replication process. To understand how this plays out, I'll attempt to explain it as simply as possible: first, recall that as long as a person's cells are dividing and replicating, then they are able to replace any damaged or dead cells in the body with another cell instead of with scar tissue, thus the person stays healthier and has the potential to live longer. For a cell to divide, it takes the two strands that make up each chromosome inside it and makes a copy of each one. This way each new cell (produced from the division) has a complete chromosome. As the enzyme that does this has to have something to grab ahold of, the part of that strand the enzyme has attached itself to will not be copied. This is where the telomeres come in—because the part of that strand the enzyme has attached itself to is the telomere.

For this replication to occur, a cell's DNA has to have—after the copying is complete—one of its two strands longer than the other. Once the replication is complete, another enzyme comes along and cuts off this longer strand. As explained in the previous paragraph, this longer strand that the enzyme attaches itself to is part of the telomere. This means that the longer strand that gets cut is part of the telomere getting cut. Consequently, the result of each cell replication is that a part of the telomere becomes shorter.

Remember, once a telomere becomes too short, cell replication can no longer happen; thus, scar tissue, a lesser substitute, is used to repair damage. In turn, this shortens each cell's life, organ's life, and, thus, the person's life. This process of cell division and shortening of the telomeres can only happen about fifty to seventy times total in the course of a lifetime. It is called the Hayflick phenomenon.[8]

The way that vitamin D3 is believed to affect aging involves this longer strand of DNA. Scientists believe that vitamin D3 prevents the cutting off of this longer strand of DNA, which means the telomere is not made shorter at this point in replication. In fact, it is at this point that an enzyme comes along and lengthens the shorter telomere, so they are both the same length as needed. As a result, the aging process slows.

Another hypothesis about vitamin D3's effect on aging, by way of DRS and also boosting the immune system, is that it works indirectly on telomeres by extending the overall life of each cell so that less replications need to occur. In this theory vitamin D3 supports cells so that they are stronger to fight infection from substances like bacteria and viruses, are less prone to damage, and promote longer lives. This means that fewer cell replications are required, and that cell replication is happening at a slower rate than in another person's body who has suboptimal levels of vitamin D3 in their blood. When cell replication is happening at a slower rate, the shortening of telomeres is also happening at a slower rate. Consequently, a person's aging slows, and they live longer. In this way, vitamin D3 isn't directly acting on telomeres to either increase their length or decrease their shortening. Instead, it's indirectly supporting telomeres by slowing cell replication, which means slowing down the rate at which telomeres must do their job.

The takeaway: although the exact mechanism isn't clear, scientists have found that vitamin D3 influences cell replication. Whether by directly affecting the length of telomeres, either keeping them longer or not shortening them, or by increasing the overall lifespan of cells, thus slowing the need for replication, vitamin D3 plays a key role in a person's aging rate. My argument and my urging: take ODA of vitamin D3, meaning 30,000 IU per day, so that your blood level reaches optimum range. When you are at COBL, meaning your vitamin D3 blood levels are in the optimum range of 100–140 ng/ml, then you allow yourself the greatest potential for slowing the aging process in your body.

Good Gene, Bad Gene: Vitamin D3 Decides

The stress the body undergoes from lack of DRS affects the body beyond accelerating the aging process. In this section, we'll look at how a lack of DRS can put such tremendous stress on the body that undesirable genes get expressed, genes that were always present but had been "silent" until thus activated or when no gene is available, the body has to try to adapt and it does so suboptimally.

Every individual's genetic makeup allows for two possibilities since there are two halves of a chromosome. Each half is from a parent, and each half is different. For every genetic pair in a chromosome, the body selects the "best" gene from the two possibilities.

The genotype is the set of genes responsible for what and how the body can function and look—so both genes contributed from each parent make up a person's genotype. The phenotype is the physical expression of that trait. Only the gene in the pair that the body selects as "best" gets expressed (at least under ideal circumstances), and this is the phenotype. The genotype can be considered the potential and the phenotype is what actually occurs.

A visual example of a genotype and a phenotype would be the following: imagine a father has red hair and the mother is blonde. The child's genotype contains both possibilities. However, if the child has red hair, then only the phenotype is red hair because this is the possibility that was expressed.

If a person has a defective gene(s), such as the genes to produce a disease (the genotype), it does not mean they will develop it (the phenotype). For example, say, you have one gene in your genotype for diabetes. That means you have the potential for diabetes. However, as long as the other half of your gene pair works great, your body selects the other good gene of the pair as "best" and expresses that as the phenotype. This means that you don't actually suffer from diabetes. In this case, it means the genotype for diabetes is not expressed (so it doesn't become a phenotype).

When the body undergoes trauma and/or stress, for reasons that aren't clear, the chosen "best" gene stops working. That phenotype goes "silent" and returns to being just a genotype. Once this happens, the less desirable gene of the pair of genes, we'll call it the "bad" gene, gets expressed, thus becomes the phenotype. In the example from the previous paragraph, this would mean that if you undergo a serious trauma or chronic stress, a result could be that the gene for diabetes, that had been "silent," gets expressed because its "good" partner gene got turned off. Or, if both of the genes were originally good copies of the gene but they became damaged, diabetes or other chronic condition could develop.

Again, the reason the body does this in response to stress and trauma isn't totally clear. However, this is what scientists have found so far: this expression of the "bad" gene is linked to the deterioration of the immune system due to trauma, stress, and/or lack of DRS (which, itself, causes stress and trauma to the body). As already explained in this chapter, during DRS, the brain and body repair, clean, and restore themselves. Vitamin D3 at optimal dosing plays a key role in the body achieving the stable state (that's when the skeletal muscles are paralyzed) necessary for these repair and cleaning processes to occur. The previous chapter covered the dependent relationship between optimal blood levels of vitamin D3 and a robust immune system. When we combine these two findings, the result is incredibly important.

Here are those findings combined: when you have optimal blood levels of vitamin D3, your immune system is primed to perform at its highest potential. Additionally, your brain is able to activate the skeletal muscle paralysis needed to keep the body stable for DRS to occur, so the needed cleaning and restoration processes can take place. The cleaning and restoration inside the brain and body also strengthen the body's immune system. In effect, optimal blood levels of vitamin D3 help a person on many levels—notably it supports the immune system via two avenues: directly and indirectly via DRS. Thus, optimal blood levels of vitamin D3 are doubly instrumental in aiding the immune system to function at its greatest capacity.

The opposite is also true: suboptimal blood levels of vitamin D3 are doubly disadvantageous to the immune system. A prolonged suboptimal level hinders both DRS and the immune system, with the potential either for activating the expression of the "bad" gene in each pair or for knocking out both good genes.

A deciding factor: vitamin D3. Optimal blood levels of vitamin D3, i.e., COBL, in the range of 100–140 ng/ml, can delay or prevent diseases like diabetes through this mechanism. Similarly, suboptimal levels make diseases like diabetes possible through this mechanism. My greatest hope is that this detailed presentation of the body's systems compels you to start a daily program of taking vitamin D3 at ODA.

Aging, Stress, and Disease

Through aging alone, the body undergoes stress. There's muscle wear and tear, which happens on the cellular level. When you combine aging with years and decades of suboptimal vitamin D3 blood levels, the body experiences even more stress. The brain and body's cells aren't able to optimally repair, restore, and clean themselves. The immune system operates at less than optimal capacity. Over time then because the body isn't able to protect itself nor repair itself as well as it could with COBL of vitamin D3, the cells, organs, and whole body breaks down faster.

This seems to best be exhibited by people who appear healthy their whole lives. Then, at a certain point, all the lack of deep restorative sleep and a less-than-optimal immune system catch up with them in a short time period. We have all seen this happen. First one ailment, say gallbladder disease, hits them. Then it's a postoperative infection, then pneumonia, and finally a heart attack. Thus, one after another, many organs fail. That is a common example of how this deterioration plays out.

Because aging puts stress on the body, with increased longevity worldwide, we see this stress- and trauma-induced expression of "bad" genes playing out. This phenomenon results in the appearance of different, new, and once-rare diseases—that is, new phenotypes—which, in the past, we didn't see. Diseases that are common killers today, like cancer, coronary heart disease, and diabetes, were rare in the past.

In the past, people didn't live as long as they do today. With their shorter lifespans, the body didn't undergo the same level of stress and trauma required to set off this expression of "bad" genes that allowed for these often-fatal diseases. Basically, people died too early for these phenomena to occur.

Let's consider the example of coronary heart disease. Until the later part of the 20th century coronary heart disease was rare. As before, most people had a shorter lifespan than people today, and they died from trauma or infections. However, with these other causes of death eliminated or incredibly reduced, people of the late 20th century to the present, on average, live much longer.

By living longer, people now have time to develop coronary artery disease because they have time for the body to age enough and undergo that particular stress and trauma that comes from age that sets off the phenomena of the unexpected expression of "bad" disease-enabling genes (or else the loss of the genes that prevent the diseases). In this way, once-rare diseases have become today's major cause of death. If not for the elimination of other causes of death and increased longevity, this would not have happened. Nor would we have come to understand the effect of coronary artery disease, nor come to understand what caused it and spent so much time and effort treating it.

The same scenario may occur in the future. What is now a rare disease could become the coronary artery disease of the future. How it would play out is that scientists and doctors would figure out how to eliminate today's commonly fatal diseases—cancer, coronary heart disease, and diabetes—so that people could live even longer. But once these diseases are eliminated, we may find a new "coronary artery-type" disease, that is, a disease that only occurs if you live to be in your 120s, for example. This would be diseases that today are considered rare, but if people are living to their 120s, these diseases would have the opportunity to get expressed more often through this "bad" gene expression mechanism.

I realize I am getting ahead of myself in presenting this possibility to you. Really, that new coronary heart-type disease of the 21st century can wait. We need to treat what is now affecting so many of us: severe obesity, sleep apnea, and type 2 diabetes, which I address in greater detail later in the book.

My reason for presenting this whole argument is simply to highlight the tremendous significance of your vitamin D3 blood level. Yes, it plays a huge role in whether you get a good night's sleep or whether you contract this year's flu. But that's not all. It also plays a leading role in whether your suppressed "bad" genes end up becoming expressed. Depending on what exactly those silent, "bad" genotypes are, this could mean the possibility that you'll be contending with diabetes, cancer, coronary heart disease, another potentially fatal disease, or a combination of crippling ailments.

The difficult part of the current most common diseases of the early 21st century is the many factors that are at play in their manifestation. The challenge is trying to connect them through a common link. It's like the trees getting in the way of seeing the forest. Though, after hearing this tired cliché for my entire life, here it fits. When we consider today's common fatal diseases—diabetes, cancer, coronary heart disease, etc.—not everyone has the same symptoms. Where one group of people with very similar genotypes has the same disease, others with similar genotypes do not. What makes it so difficult to put together is the individuals experiencing them may have different reactions.

Chapter Recap

Deep restorative sleep (DRS) is incredibly important in your daily wellbeing and long-term health. It's the time when the brain and body repairs, replenishes, and restores itself. Your vitamin D3 blood level plays a key role in your body's ability to achieve DRS—or not. Optimal vitamin D3 blood levels signal the brain to put the body in muscle paralysis during the REM stage of the sleep cycle. This paralysis keeps you from thrashing about and waking yourself up, which would interrupt the all-important brain and body maintenance that happens during REM. However, when your vitamin D3 levels are suboptimal, the necessary muscle paralysis isn't achieved, so you wake many times in the night (perhaps you mistakenly believe it's because you have to urinate), and DSR sleep doesn't happen, REM sleep doesn't happen either or gets interrupted, and the body and brain don't get the needed maintenance. Over time, this can open the door to unwanted diseases mental and physical, and to accelerated aging. As many research studies have found (even at the suboptimal levels of vitamin D3 their subjects were taking), there is a connection between vitamin D and sleep, with the greater doses of vitamin D correlating to longer and better sleep.

The big chapter takeaway: take ODA of vitamin D3 to achieve the necessary level of vitamin D3 in your blood to optimally position yourself to get deep restorative sleep and the many optimal health and wellbeing benefits that come with it.

Next Up

If you've tried many diets and had little to no success, in the next chapter you'll learn that it was not due to a lack of willpower or weakness on your part. It's due to winter syndrome. The next chapter dissects how vitamin D3 and obesity connect and offers a solution to those struggling to lose weight. Plus, chapter 7 addresses vitamin D3 and type 2 diabetes.

Chapter 6 Notes

1. W.E. Stumpf and L.P. O'Brien, "1,25 (OH)2 Vitamin D3 Sites of Action in the Brain. An Autoradiographic Study," *Histochemistry* 87, no. 5 (June 17, 1987): 393–406.

2. "Brain Basics: Understanding sleep," from National Institute of Neurological Disorders and Stroke, last modified July 6, 2018, accessed September 17, 2018, https://www.ninds.nih.gov/Disorders/Patient-Caregiver-Education/Understanding-Sleep.

3. M.S. Majid et al. "The Effect of Vitamin D Supplement on the Score and Quality of Sleep in 20–50 Year-old People with Sleep Disorders Compared with Control Group," *Nutritional Neuroscience* 21, no. 7 (September 2018): 511– 519, doi: 10.1080/1028415X.2017.1317395

4. J. Massa et al. "Vitamin D and Actigraphic Sleep Outcomes in Older Community-Dwelling Men: The MrOS Sleep Study," *Sleep* 38 no. 2, (February 1, 2015): 251–257, https://doi.org/10.5665/sleep.4408.

5. J.H. Kim et al. "Clinical Investigations Association Between Self-Reported Sleep Duration and Serum Vitamin D Level in Elderly Korean Adults," *Journal of the American Geriatrics Society* 62, no 12. (December 2014): 2327–2332, https://doi.org/10.1111/jgs.13148.

6. S.M. Bertisch, "25-Hydroxyvitamin D Concentration and Sleep Duration and Continuity: Multi-Ethnic Study of Atherosclerosis," *Sleep* 38, no. 8 (August 1, 2015): 1305–1311, https://doi.org/10.5665/sleep.4914.

7. S. Daniells, "Higher Vitamin D Levels Linked to Longer Telomeres: Study," Nutra Ingredients-USA, February 10, 2017, accessed September 17, 2018, https://www.nutraingredients-usa.com/Article/2017/02/10/Higher-vitamin-D-levels-linked-to-longer-telomeres-Study.

8. L. Hayflick and P.S. Moorehead, "Serial Cultivation of Human Diploid Cell Strains," *Experimental Cell Research* 25 no. 3 (December 1961): 585–621.

Chapter 7

Vitamin D3, Metabolic Activity, and Weight Loss

Like so many Americans, I and many of my patients were struggling with obesity, that is, until we began taking ODA of vitamin D3 and our vitamin D3 blood levels reached COBL. Once this happened, our eating and weight problems changed. I'll explain by telling the stories of three patients—Marina, David, and Rafael (all pseudonyms)—as well as my own story. After their stories, we'll look at what's going on in the body with vitamin D3 that resulted in these changes.

Marina weighed 350 pounds when she first started taking ODA of vitamin D3. As Marina is five feet, six inches in height, her ideal body weight is around 150 pounds. To calculate a woman's ideal body weight, the base is a hundred pounds for the first five feet in height. Then you add five pounds for every inch above. This is an accepted method for giving an approximation of a typical woman's ideal body weight.

Once at COBL, Marina was losing about ten pounds a month. After the first month she was at 340 pounds. The next month 330 pounds, etc. All the while, Marina visited my office once a month, so we could monitor her vitamin D3 and calcium levels. Because these losses were subtle and happened over time, when I saw Marina each month I didn't detect from her appearance that she'd lost weight. However, she would tell me at each visit that she'd lost another ten pounds. Her weigh-ins and charts, of course, made record of this. Two-and-a-half years into COBL and once-a-month blood checks, Marina now weighs in at 150 pounds.

"Dr. Somerville, remember when I was 350 pounds 2.5 years ago?" Marina commented to me.

I was floored. Surprisingly, I'd forgotten because Marina's weight loss had been so slow, steady, and prolonged.

In these years, Marina hadn't taken any fat blocking medicines, received no bariatric surgery, and was on no special diets or exercise regimens. As she explained it, "Really, my appetite changed."

Before, she would eat a huge amount of food and still be very hungry, but then her appetite shifted. Once her vitamin D3 blood levels were at COBL, that's when she noticed this shift.

Let me add that Marina's weight has settled around 135 pounds. She continues to take vitamin D3 at ODA.

Unlike Marina, David and Rafael were not morbidly obese, but they were certainly overweight. Each of these men was five feet, eight inches tall and weighed 245 and 250 pounds, respectively. The accepted ideal body weight for men is calculated at 120 pounds for the first five feet in height. Then you add seven pounds for each inch beyond that. David and Rafael's ideal body weight would be in the area of 176 pounds.

When David and Rafael respectively began taking ODA of vitamin D3, they ended up losing weight at an incredibly rapid pace: twenty-five pounds per month. After three months, both had lost seventy-five pounds, and thus had reached their approximate ideal body weights of about 175 pounds. That's where their weight stabilized.

Losing weight at that kind of rate, twenty-five pounds a month, is not recommended because it puts a lot of stress on the body. However, both men reported that they didn't feel as if they were suffering during the three months. Each actually commented that they felt great the whole time. They each noted that similar to what Marina said, they didn't actively go on a diet plan or an exercise regimen. Instead, they were less hungry than before, less hungry and notably more energetic. They didn't feel like sitting around so much and found themselves up and doing things while at the same time their appetites were satisfied with less food as compared to before. They were also sleeping so much better. Wow! What's going on?

Let me tell you about myself and then we'll go into what's going on. Up until I had my cycling accident, I'd been an avid exerciser. But after the accident, confined to a wheelchair and also finishing my residency, moving back to Texas and starting my own practice, as well as being a father and husband, my exercise became minimal. My sun exposure was minimal. I was working a lot—and as you know from earlier chapters—my sleep quality became very poor as was the state of my immune system. On top of this I was very hungry. I could eat a lot, I put on weight, but I still felt hungry and kept eating.

Once I learned about vitamin D3, increased my daily intake to 30,000 IU per day, and later my blood level of vitamin D3 became optimal, I too noticed a shift in my appetite. I became increasingly less hungry and more satisfied with smaller and smaller portions of food. Over two years, I ended up losing around one hundred pounds, and I've maintained that weight loss to this day—that's six years later and counting.

Admittedly, these examples of weight loss from Marina, David, Rafael, and myself—are very impressive. What appeared more typical among my patients taking ODA of vitamin D3 was each patient losing around ten pounds per month. Patients who were underweight ended up gaining weight. Besides losing weight, some of my patients also lost diseases, most prominently type 2 diabetes—something we'll look at later in this chapter.

So what's going on? Why this shift in appetite once our blood levels of vitamin D3 were optimal? Why this weight loss? For that matter, when blood levels are suboptimal, why is the appetite for food so great?

Vitamin D3 as a Metabolic Hormone

To explain what's going on we start by looking at how the body and our diet interact. Although we, human beings, have made tremendous advances in technology, the sciences, the arts, and more, and despite our ability to think and reason, the body's hormonal systems remain primitive. For our ancestors, centuries and millennia before us, the hormonal systems worked well, protecting them from themselves, as I'll soon lay out. But for us modern humans, the lives we live don't necessarily match the primitive conditions our hormonal systems assume we are living under.

To clarify, the body has many hormonal pathways. One hormone, like vitamin D3, doesn't play a role in a single pathway. It's much more complex than that. Thus far in this book, we've discussed how vitamin D3 plays a hormonal role in several systems: the calcium/phosphate balance, the immune system and, in particular, the gut, and the activation of skeletal muscle paralysis in the brain during sleep. Therefore, you can see vitamin D3 plays multiple important roles in a variety of processes in the body. Here, we're looking at how vitamin D3 plays an important role in another hormonal system—how it relates to metabolism, appetite, and fat absorption. What you'll soon see too is how, at suboptimal levels, the lack of vitamin D3's hormonal effects lead to winter syndrome.

The hormonal system that we're focusing on is the one that keeps us alive, protected, and in sync with the seasons. For, in times past, when most human beings, in the Northern and Southern Hemispheres especially, lived according to the seasons, if they depended on their rational thoughts over the signals their bodies were giving them, then they might make poor decisions that would cause them and their children to die of starvation, infection, or cold. Instead, it was the levels of the hormone vitamin D3 in their blood and bodies that essentially, acted upon them internally to make important season-related decisions. Consequently, because their hormones were moving them, they didn't have to make active decisions, which could prove fatal. To explain what I mean, let's look at an illustration.

Let's consider a bear—a mammal that also developed a similar vitamin D3 hormonal system for signaling the seasons (except bears, like other fur-covered animals, produce vitamin D3 from UVB light in a way that's different from humans because, unlike humans, their skin isn't exposed to sunlight; it's mostly covered in fur). To briefly and simply explain it, substances on the bear's fur are converted to vitamin D3 by UVB, so when a bear grooms itself, it ingests the vitamin D3. The bear actually experiences a "craving" for the vitamin D3, and it stimulates it to seek sunlight and lick its fur. Let's imagine a bear in Toronto, Canada, in January, where the average temperature is below freezing. This bear is in hibernation. This means it is in a state of inactivity for several months, with low body temperature, slow breathing and heart rate, and a low metabolic rate.

Now imagine that something strange happens with the weather, and there are three days at 90 degrees Fahrenheit. Based on the air temperature of these three days, the bear might figure that summer is here, so it should come out of hibernation—that is, if the bear relied on its brain to make active decisions in this regard.

However, that's not the way such an important decision happens. In fact, it's the bear's hormonal system that signals the bear to come out of hibernation or not. Even with three hot days in the middle of winter, the bear's vitamin D blood levels are not at the correct level to indicate winter is over. Thus, the bear's body knows it is too early to come out of hibernation.

Even if the bear left its den, its body would detect that it's too early to emerge from hibernation, even if the air temperature is high. In Canada in January, the sun angle is low and the amount of sunlight (the UVB type to produce vitamin D3) available during the day is either absent or comparatively not much. Also, there are approximately eight hours of daylight in the winter in Toronto and seventeen in the summer, which the bear may notice. Consequently, if the bear emerged, its body wouldn't take in the appropriate levels of UVB rays that would produce vitamin D3 at the "spring-time" levels (because spring is when mammals do come out of hibernation).

The bear's body knows on two levels that it should remain in hibernation: both its current low blood level of vitamin D3 and the very little amount or lack of sunlight (UVB), thus vitamin D3, it receives if it emerges. Hormones, in this case vitamin D3, use the more reliable production of vitamin D3—not air temperature—to signal to the bear when to come out of hibernation (and for that matter, when to go into it). Thus, the vitamin D3 hormone protects the bear from potentially faulty reasoning.

As with bears and other mammals, in human bodies as well, vitamin D3 acts hormonally to signal the season changes. Increasing blood levels are consistent with spring and summer in which the very increased vitamin D3 levels signal summer, decreasing levels signal the fall, and finally very low levels signal winter, and then finally increasing levels signal spring. Thus, vitamin D3 tells us the seasons and is our hormonal clock. It's a slow and steady but stable mechanism that developed as a way of protecting human beings. It allows us to better survive our environments, especially those with seasonal changes in food availability. Of course, this mechanism becomes problematic when humans are not exposed to the natural patterns of the sun and those patterns no longer equate to food availability. That's where we modern humans are.

Hormonal Signaling, Seasons, and Food Availability

As already noted, the summertime, with its consistent and prolonged days of sunlight in the Northern and Southern Hemispheres, is also when the human body produces its top levels of vitamin D3. While the body stores excess vitamin D3 for the coming dark months, in terms of vitamin D3's hormonal signaling during the summertime it increases the metabolism up to twenty to thirty percent from wintertime levels. It increases overall energy levels. It decreases the appetite. And it decreases the small intestines' absorption (thus, storing) of fat and instead encourages the body to expend as energy any fat taken in from food.

It makes sense that vitamin D3 blood levels set this in motion in the summertime because summertime is the time of year when food availability is at its highest. With its regular and prolonged days of sunlight in the Northern and Southern Hemispheres, plants are at their most lush and robust. Fruits, vegetables, seeds, and nuts are aplenty. This vegetation provides a cornucopia of food for humans and all animals. Whether it is plant-based or animal-based foods, summer is the time when food is plentiful. Sugar, fat, and protein are aplenty. The body's metabolic response, as activated by the vitamin D3 hormone, is reflective of this.

In wintertime, a time that food, traditionally is scarce, the body's metabolic response, as activated by the vitamin D3 hormone, is reflective of that scarcity. We, of course, know that humans don't hibernate in the winter as do bears and many other mammals. However, the very little vitamin D3 available from the short daylight hours combined with the ever-decreasing levels of vitamin D3 in the blood (as acquired and stored from the summer months) signal the human body that food is scarce and the body should conserve what little it comes across. Accordingly, to fight starvation the metabolism slows, twenty to thirty percent slower than that of summer. The appetite increases and changes, so that if we do come across food, we are driven to consume as much of it as possible. Our appetite changes in that we now crave calorie-rich foods—think potatoes and gravy, or cinnamon buns. And our fat absorption increases, meaning on the off chance we consume a fatty food, the body will store it, as opposed to burning it off as energy.

The body's internal hormonal signal makes sense considering food scarcity in the winter—at least in times past. The winter, with its low sun angle in the sky, low or no UVB, and typically colder temperatures means no new vegetation, thus much less plant- and animal-based food availability. The body interprets the lower vitamin D3 blood levels and the long period of insufficient UVB, and makes those internal changes described in the previous paragraph—all to ensure people's survival.

The Unappeasable Appetite

In the way most people in the modern world live, especially people in developed countries like the USA, the seasonal hormonal effect has gone off the rails. There is a total mismatch between the metabolic responses our vitamin D3 blood levels are activating and the actual "season" we find ourselves in. The result: the current obesity epidemic.

As already detailed in chapter 4, most of us in the developed world neither live according to the seasons, nor are we exposed much to the sun. For the most part, our jobs have regular schedules that aren't dependent on the season. A lot of these jobs take place inside buildings, indoors. In this way we aren't getting a lot of sunlight in the summer and very little in the winter. Instead, all year long, we get fairly low levels of sunlight (thus, we maintain suboptimal blood levels of vitamin D3). On top of that, because of the link between sun exposure and skin cancer and accelerated skin aging, avoiding the sun is a common practice for many people, using sunscreen, sunblock, hats, and protective clothing. This also contributes to most people's sustained suboptimal blood levels of vitamin D3.

Again, as already explained, suboptimal blood levels of vitamin D3 over a prolonged period result in a condition that I've dubbed winter syndrome. Winter syndrome entails a poorly responsive immune system (chapter 4), a chronic lack of deep restorative sleep (DRS; chapter 5), and a mismatched metabolism (current chapter). Let's explore the mismatched metabolism.

Because most of us in the developed world in the Northern and Southern Hemispheres have such low blood levels of vitamin D3, our bodies assume it is winter—all year long. Accordingly, to make sure we survive the winter when food is so scarce, our appetites are increased and changed so that we crave the most calorically-dense foods possible and a lot of it. Second our metabolism slows by twenty to thirty percent to increase conversion of excess food intake into fat. Finally, it results in our small intestines working full throttle in absorbing the fats and excess calories from the rich foods we've been signaled to consume. Then our bodies are super efficient in storing that excess as fat on our bodies.

I call this a "mismatched" metabolism because not only is it not winter all year long, but in today's developed world, we don't deal with food scarcity, neither in the winter nor any other time of year. In fact, all year long, in developed countries at least, most people have more than enough fatty, sugary, and protein-rich foods available to them. So, all year long our food availability is like that of summertime, but our bodies are interacting with food as if they are in a scarcity state. Hence—the tragic mismatch, the result of which is winter syndrome.

The mismatch is tragic in that the body's seasonal hormonal effect developed as a way to protect people and increase their likelihood of survival. However, because that same system has determined that we are in a perpetual winter, when in fact our food reality is more like a perpetual summer, it is doing all it can to ensure we put on more and more weight, that we are fat, ravenous, and ever-gaining weight. It's like someone who vigilantly wears their seatbelt, but then rather than protecting them, it is because of the seatbelt that they get seriously injured or killed in a car accident. It's a mismatch, and it's tragic. And it is a huge contributing factor in our current obesity epidemic. Of course, other factors are at play as well—an overabundance of cheap food that is highly caloric but low in nutrients and food addiction. Even still, I argue that the major contributing factor to the current obesity epidemic is our chronic sub-optimal blood levels of vitamin D3 such that our body positions itself on the inside to prepare for food scarcity, a condition I call winter syndrome.

From this explanation of what's going on inside the body, our ravenous appetite—even after we've eaten plenty of food—suddenly makes sense. Our hormones are telling us food is scarce, so no matter how much we take in, the body demands that we take in more. Accordingly, we have huge appetites.

With this explanation our struggles and eventual failures with diets upon diets suddenly makes sense. When a person goes on a diet and cuts their calorie consumption, the body, which was already working as if it was in a time of food scarcity (due to winter syndrome), panics. Rather than shedding excess weight, when a dieter cuts calories, the body slows the metabolism even more, so that little or no weight is lost, or so that weight is gained from the fewer calories that are consumed. Hence, the person on the diet feels like they failed, so they stop—only to try again later on, but the cycle repeats. Why? Because the whole time, the person has winter syndrome; hence, their body is primed for food scarcity.

The solution: optimal dosing of vitamin D3 to get the body out of winter syndrome and get the body's metabolic responses in line with the vast food available to us all year long in our modern lives. Optimal blood levels of vitamin D3 equate to the blood levels humans historically experienced in the summer, the very time of year when food sources, traditionally, were at the most abundant—which parallels our current food availability all year long: summer-like abundance all year long, no matter the season, at least for most of us living in developed countries.

As testified by Marina, David, Rafael, and me in the opening of this chapter, with optimal blood levels of vitamin D3, your appetite slowly and steadily adjusts downward. You no longer crave rich and caloric foods to maximize the amount of fat storage. The appetite is quickly satiated with less food. In fact, your appetite matches only what you need or possibly even less. For example, if, like most Americans, you have excess fat, once you are at optimal blood levels of vitamin D3, those fat deposits start a flow in the opposite direction—they get burned up as energy—which makes sense because optimal blood levels of vitamin D3 are signaling the body that food is abundant and scarcity isn't a problem.

In fact, once at optimal levels of vitamin D3, until the body fat levels are reduced to ideal levels, your food consumption will decrease below what is needed. This burning off of fat is assisted by the metabolism increasing twenty to thirty percent. Again, this is in keeping with those high, summertime levels of vitamin D3, which COBL matches. Also, fat absorption shrinks drastically to only the necessary fats. The body has no need to store fat because its internal vitamin D3 signaling indicates that there's plenty of food available.

When you are at COBL of vitamin D3, whereas before you could eat a large plate of food and still be hungry, now you eat a small plate of food and that's enough. You don't want or need more as you are not hungry. You no longer are hungry for seconds or thirds. Your three regular, normal-sized meals are fine.

Perhaps you are thinking, "Wait—if I take optimal doses of vitamin D3 and it changes my appetite, what exactly does that mean? Does it mean food is going to taste like cardboard? That I will no longer enjoy eating?" The answer: no not at all. It only means that eating one steak is enough. Yes, it still tastes the same, but, no, you don't have to eat several to be satiated.

This should make sense to you because when the vitamin D3 in your blood is at optimal levels, then your body is no longer in a food-scarcity mode. It's not protecting you from starvation. At optimal levels, your body is in summer mode, ready to be active and with no fear of scarcity. Your body at optimal levels matches its internal responses to the current high food availability that is the norm for most of us in developed countries.

Fat Absorption and Vitamin D3

The third and perhaps most important effect of optimal dosing and optimal blood levels of vitamin D3 is its effect on our fat absorption, something touched on already. Let's dive into it more fully.

For a while, all the rage to lose weight was pharmaceutical fat blockers. These are prescription medications and what I call "imitation" fat blockers. These medications blocked the small intestine from absorbing a percentage of the fats consumed in food. Instead, fats simply passed through and were excreted as waste in bowel movements. However, because some had serious side effects—damaging the heart valves—many were pulled from the market.

The serious side effects aside, I view fat blockers as incredibly flawed because they only addressed one variable—blocking fat absorption—in inciting weight loss. In a way, fat blockers could be seen as encouraging bad eating habits like seriously gorging yourself because the fat blockers would allow you to expel much of the food without "paying the penalty," so to speak, of gaining weight. On top of this, the body actually needs many fats to function in an optimal matter, so blocking fat absorption, I would suspect, is dangerous. In this way, those fat blockers shared a similarity with bariatric surgery, which results in deficiencies of vitamins and minerals. Over the long term, this can't be healthy. Also, they do nothing to alter appetite nor increase metabolic rate like optimal blood levels of vitamin D3 do.

As I see it, vitamin D3 at optimal doses is the ideal "weight loss drug" because it addresses three different factors: minimizing fat absorption in the small intestine, increasing the metabolism by twenty to thirty percent, and decreasing the appetite. On top of this, vitamin D3 isn't a new compound developed in a lab. It's a hormone that the body can produce on its own. Taking it in optimal doses in supplement form is more natural and simpler than taking a chemist-created and patented pharmaceutical. Vitamin D3 does not try and trick the body. Optimal dosing of vitamin D3, in fact, puts the body and mind into a more normal balance.

Type 2 Diabetes

Diabetes is in and of itself a huge problem globally affecting 135 million in 1995 and expected to effect 300 million by 2025.[1] Most people who suffer diabetes suffer from type 2. Those with type 2 diabetes have a similar physical appearance, what I describe as classic winter syndrome physical effects: obesity that's usually severe as well as dark circles with puffiness under their eyes.

People with type 2 diabetes often have insatiable appetites. Also, they typically have all the sleep issues discussed in chapter 5 as well as the other issues associated with suboptimal dosing of vitamin D3.

Type 2 diabetes is an acquired disease, meaning one a person contracts after birth usually by a disease-causing agent or from lifestyle choices. Type 2 diabetes is reversible. It's theorized that type 2 diabetes results from a person gaining so much weight, such that their insulin secretion is not enough to meet their body's needs or the cells are so resistant that the body cannot secret enough insulin. Both of these are mechanisms for type 2 diabetes. Consequently, often just by losing weight, a person can either lose or greatly improve their diabetes. This has been shown to happen by those who have bariatric surgery and lose weight (though after this surgery some have their diabetes resolve without their losing weight. This indicates that with bariatric surgery something else is going on too, but what that is is not yet clear). Diabetes is one of the often-cited reasons to have this type of surgery.[2] Yes, there are other effects that this type of surgery has on the small intestine and gut flora, but these are also where optimal levels of vitamin D3 come into effect.[3] Again, more study is needed.

I practiced medicine in Texas along the border of Mexico. In my region diabetes is an epidemic. Many of my patients have type 2 diabetes. What's happened is that many of my diabetic patients have discovered that after they start optimal dosing, once their blood level of vitamin D3 has reached COBL, they need less—and sometimes much, much less—of the blood sugar lowering medications than they were previously taking. Let me give you some examples, and then we'll explore what's going on in the body when blood levels are at COBL that allow for this.

My patient, let's call him Joshua, was a very brittle diabetic. A brittle diabetic is one who needs lots of insulin to lower their blood sugar, and it does not take much sugar intake to spike their blood sugar. Soon after Joshua started taking 30,000 IUs of vitamin D3 a day, he noticed that in the morning he was light headed and sweaty. Upon doing a finger stick blood sugar test, he discovered that, indeed, his blood sugar was low. He'd had the opposite issue before. In checking his blood sugar before taking ODA, it was always high in the morning.

When Joshua reported this to me, to be safe I had him stop taking the vitamin D3. Joshua already had an appointment to see his general doctor who was managing his diabetes the next day. I advised Joshua to discuss his new symptoms with his other doctor. After speaking with his other doctor, that doctor lowered Joshua's evening insulin dose. Next, Joshua restarted the vitamin D3 as I directed. His morning sweats and other symptoms of low blood sugar from too much insulin resolved, and with the optimal blood levels of vitamin D3 he needed less insulin each day.

Joshua was the first of many cases that alerted me to the fact that vitamin D3 affects the blood sugar levels of those who are diabetic. My plan with the patients was that they inform the doctors' managing their diabetic medications that they were starting optimal dosing of vitamin D3 and that it could be necessary to lower their diabetic medications levels.

I had another patient, Trevor (a pseudonym) who was taking over 270 units of insulin a day. Trevor was able to cut back his dose by 100 units a day. This was an extreme example of the positive effect of vitamin D3 at ODA. Of course, every patient is different, but it further demonstrated to me there was something beyond placebo going on.

If you are a diabetic, like with my patients, it is important that you discuss optimal dosing with the physician who is managing your diabetes before you begin taking vitamin D3. If they are not open to discussing it, then you have to decide if they are open-minded and doing what's best for you—or not.

Joshua and Trevor are examples of patients with very severe diabetes whose severity greatly decreased due to vitamin D3 at COBL. There were many other patients who were only mild diabetics and required low doses of oral diabetic medications for treatment. With time as they maintained COBL they were able to stop these medications completely. This was under my and their doctors' care, and not something to do without professional help. This makes sense.

So what is going on with vitamin D3 to affect diabetes? As already laid out, the body with COBL vitamin D3 while consuming ODA of vitamin D3 is now able to improve its metabolic function: by increasing the metabolism by twenty to thirty percent; by absorbing less fats; and by decreasing the appetite such that foods high in sugars and fats are no longer the main craving.

When these metabolic changes occur, one result is a reduction in blood sugar levels. There are several avenues that the reduction in blood sugar might occur:

- When vitamin D3 increases the metabolism, this results in the burning of more sugar. Hence, blood sugar levels are reduced.

- Vitamin D3 may instigate the small intestine to absorb less sugar in the first place and simply pass the rest for excretion. Hence, blood sugar levels are reduced.

- Vitamin D3, as noted in chapter 4, affects the intestinal flora such that the propagation of helpful gut flora abounds. This flora might consume sugar (before it reaches the intestines where it is absorbed into the blood), which in turn reduces the amount of sugar that is absorbed into the blood.

- Another idea is that with the body at optimal dosing and optimal blood levels of vitamin D3, there is less fat absorbed. Thus, more of the calories to run basic metabolic function will come from proteins or sugars. Since both are less than half as caloric as fat, it requires a lot more by weight of both. At ODA the body ends up using and burning more sugar, which results in a reduction in blood sugar levels.

- Because fats affect the ability of insulin to interact with cells, another possibility is that at COBL there's less fat in the bloodstream. This, in turn, could make insulin more effective at balancing blood sugar levels.

- Also, when a person loses weight, the body's insulin has fewer cells to work with, so it can be more effective in driving the sugar out of the blood and into the cells.

- The final possibility is that just as optimal dosing of vitamin D3 alters a person's appetite for fats, optimal dosing of vitamin D3 may do the same for sugars. The change of appetite though may be more general in that it generally decreases the appetite for everything, including sugars, which would result in decreased blood sugar levels.

By one, some, or all of these routes (the mechanism needs to be studied), there is less sugar in circulation, thus, a reduction in a person's blood sugar level. It should be noted that this change in blood sugar takes time.

Again, if you are a diabetic, consult the doctor managing your diabetes about optimal dosing of vitamin D3 before beginning.

Chapter Recap

You now understand why your body wasn't cooperating when you've tried and failed to lose weight in the past. You know too that it wasn't because you are weak or lack willpower. It was due to winter syndrome, something you can reverse by taking ODA of vitamin D3.

Optimal dosing of vitamin D3 reduces fat absorption in the small intestine, increases the metabolism twenty to thirty percent, and alters the appetite such that you start reverting into your summer body. Winter syndrome and its associated diseases, the result of prolonged vitamin D deficiency, will stop progressing and in some ways resolve. By combining optimal dosing, working with your doctor, and a reasonable long-term healthy diet, regular exercise, and support from friends and family, you should be able to take the weight off and keep it off. Don't fear the notion of a "reasonable long-term healthy diet" because COBL of vitamin D3 instigates those key metabolic changes such that eating healthy no longer becomes a struggle. You'll feel great, lose weight, look great, and save money on food and medicines.

Next Up

The final chapter of this book offers a review of all you've learned about vitamin D3 and its effects on your health. Use this conclusion chapter to recall what a vastly important role vitamin D3 plays in your health and to provide you any final motivation on why it's crucial that you start taking 30,000 IU of vitamin D3 today to get your blood levels to optimal and position yourself to be in optimal health.

Chapter 7 Notes

1. K.M.V. Narayan et al. "Diabetes—A Common Growing, Serious, Costly and Potentially Preventable Public Health Problem," *Diabetes Research and Clinical Practice* 50, Supplement 2, (October 2000): S77–S84.

2. W.T. Cefalu, F. Rubino, and D.E. Cummings, "Metabolic Surgery for Type 2 Diabetes: Changing the Landscape of Diabetes Care," *Diabetes Care* 39, no. 6 (June 2016): 857–860, https://doi.org/10.2337/dc16-0686.

3. F. Rubino and J. Marescaux, "The Effect of Duodenal-Jejunal Exclusion in Non-obese Animal Model of Type 2 Diabetes: A New Perspective for an Old Disease," *Annals of Surgery* 239, no. 1 (January 2004): 1–11.

Chapter 8

Out of the Cold and Into the Summer Sun: Optimal Dosing

In closing, let's revisit the major stops on our epic journey from a state of perpetual winter and disintegrating health to that of summer where our bodies, spirits, and minds are at their optimal.

We started with the story of my own persistent and desperate search for some kind of relief both for my own and many of my patients' chronic lack of deep restorative sleep. It was upon hearing Dr. Stasha Gominak's presentation at a medical conference that I first learned about taking vitamin D3 at doses far above the RDA of vitamin D3, 600 IU. Based upon her recommendations and the results I found for myself and my patients, I landed on 30,000 IU as the optimal daily administration (ODA) of vitamin D3. It's this ODA that allows you to achieve and maintain the clinical optimal blood level (COBL) of 100–140 ng/ml of vitamin D3. When your blood level of vitamin D3 is at COBL, you position yourself to receive the optimal benefits vitamin D3 has to offer—an optimal state of health I have named Madison-HannaH effects.

For the past eight years and counting, I have been taking ODA of vitamin D3 as have a few thousand of my patients, and we have moved from winter syndrome to Madison-HannaH effects. We have experienced significant improvements in our overall health. In fact, I believe I am alive, close to one hundred pounds lighter, and sleeping like a baby, due to optimal dosing of vitamin D3. Those patients and I have seen our quality of life vastly improved with much less illness, more energy, and less personal struggle each day.

Considering the multifaceted role vitamin D3 has played in the human body for millennia, this positive change in our health due to vitamin D3 ODA actually makes sense. As detailed in chapter 5, 6, and 7, vitamin D3 plays key roles in positioning the immune system, brain (for sleep), and metabolism to function most effectively. When your blood level of vitamin D3 is at COBL, you are primed to optimize your immune system's capabilities, which will help protect you from seasonal viruses like the flu. When your blood level of vitamin D3 is at COBL, your brain is positioned to trigger skeletal muscle paralysis needed to achieve deep restorative sleep, during which your brain and body clean, restore, and heal themselves. When your blood level of vitamin D3 is at COBL, then your metabolism is primed to work at its optimum, such that there's a reduction in fat absorption, an increase in the metabolic rate, and a decrease in appetite.

When vitamin D3 is at COBL and can play out its key roles in the systems of the body to the fullest, the trickle down effects from a strong immune system, regular deep restorative sleep, and an optimal functioning metabolic system are many. Let's look at those benefits again.

Optimal dosing of vitamin D3 helps to:

- eliminate sleep apnea,
- eliminate restless leg syndrome,
- restore deep restorative sleep,
- allow you to wake up rested and full of energy,
- prevent or eliminate snoring,
- resolve allergies,
- eliminate influenza,
- correct autism spectrum disorder,
- slow or eliminate dementia,
- slow or eliminate Alzheimer's disease,
- prevent Lyme disease and other viral diseases,
- prevent cancer,

- extend your life if you do have cancer,
- fight off TB,
- restore your ideal body weight, which for many involves the loss of massive amounts of weight,
- change your appetite, so you are easily satiated and not craving food,
- block unneeded and excess fat absorption (most),
- boost metabolism 20–30%,
- boost muscle strength 30–40%,
- increase fertility,
- boost energy 20–30%,
- slow aging,
- close and heal chronic wounds,
- fight off bacterial infections like MRSA,
- prevent diabetes,
- prevent multiple sclerosis,
- fight off any of the above listed diseases, and
- boost the immune system.

As my patients and I have found, there is not much that optimal dosing of vitamin D3 won't do to improve your life.

With such a low risk, why wouldn't you give it a try? It just might save your life and the lives of those you care about.

By adopting ODA you can start to reverse the effects of the decades of inadequate vitamin D intake on your body. You can change your body from its winter state to its summer state and reap all the benefits the summer state offers. Start ODA vitamin D3 today, so you can protect yourself from chronic sleep deprivation, obesity, and feelings of helplessness.

While modernization, mechanization, and technological and scientific breakthroughs have given people so much and changed our lives and behaviors often for the better, the resulting sun avoidance has come at a great cost. Our vitamin D levels are at a suboptimal state, and as a result we're enduring winter syndrome and we don't even realize it.

Simply by taking ODA of vitamin D3, thus taking in as supplements vitamin D3 amounts our ancestors managed to get from exposure to the summer sun, we can emerge from this winter. We can position ourselves to experience Madison-HannaH effects and the many health benefits that come with it.

Optimal dosing of vitamin D3 works. It's had a continuing positive effect on me as well as thousands of patients under my care. Prevention is better than treatment. Put your best foot forward for your own health and wellbeing today by making ODA of vitamin D3 a part of your daily routine. The alternative is maintaining the status quo, which is resulting in millions and perhaps tens of millions of premature deaths a year.

Hopefully this book will stimulate debate on this subject to start studies with vitamin D3 dosing and blood levels that make sense and that verify the significant results I and thousands of others who followed my recommendations have found. Granted, my experience is with only a select part of the population in South Texas, but I believe these results are applicable worldwide.

Please check out my website www.vitamindblog.com for further information and future books. On my site you'll find a place where you can post questions, comments, and give me progress reports in regard to how ODA of vitamin D3 is changing your health to the optimum. You too can join the thousands of my patients who are optimizing their health by optimal dosing of vitamin D3.

Appendix:

Some of My Patients' Experiences with Vitamin D3 Optimal Dosing

From Lewis Wagner in Laredo, Texas

Seven-plus years ago I had major reconstructive surgery on my right knee. I was on a bunch of pain medications, couldn't sleep, and was gaining weight. And most importantly, I couldn't interact with my children and be a dad. I was not active, so I couldn't wrestle and play with them. I was in free fall and becoming depressed.

I had played sports my whole life—soccer, football, and baseball. Going from such an active, athletic life style to suddenly having none was difficult for me. I was spinning out of control into depression and an ugly state—mentally and physically.

In addition, I was overweight at 240 pounds. This made me feel horrible. Horrible. Plus, I started snoring. And I was waking up four to six times a night, mostly due to my painful knee.

I was getting sick a lot during this time, often two times a month. I was in a downward spiral and feeling worse every day.

I started to have heart issues.

To make matters worse, my wife started feeling horrible as well, having many of my same issues.

One of my friends recommended that I see Dr. Somerville who had helped him in the past. During my first visit with Dr. Somerville, he told me flat out that I needed to take care of my wellness, and he wasn't afraid of trying new things. He told me straight up what to do. He wasn't playing games. For the first time ever, I recognized that this doctor cared! He wanted me to improve and not keep charging me for his "practicing." I knew straightaway he was a man of compassion, really helping others and making them well, so they did not have to come back and spend more money with him. He wanted me well and my wellness back.

Boy, did it feel good to meet a doctor like that!

Dr. Somerville first got me off of my addictive pain pills and tried to help me sleep better. I have a very high titration level, meaning I can handle stronger drugs. My pain threshold is off the chart. Because of this, no medication was working.

Seven-plus years ago, Dr. Somerville started me on vitamin D3 supplements. I was game, as I wanted to try anything that might work. He told me he had been giving vitamin D3 to his patients and getting good results. He recommended I start taking optimal doses of vitamin D3. So, I did it.

Almost immediately, within days, I was sleeping better. I then discovered that I was more rested, had more bounce in my step, and had more energy. I started thinking better. It was like a light bulb in my body went off and told my body, "OK. Everything is fine now." I became more thoughtful and able to concentrate at work.

Because I was so shocked at these quick results, I started to do my own research. I couldn't believe that this over-the-counter supplement was having such a great impact on my life and wellness.

Within six weeks I started to notice weight loss—but I hadn't changed my eating habits, at least not intentionally. In the first four months I lost twenty-two pounds. And let me say I was not working out at all as I was too busy and didn't have the time.

After four months I inadvertently missed a few days of taking optimal doses of the supplement. You see, I ran out and simply forgot to buy more vitamin D3 supplements. Within two days, I noticed that I felt different, like my body was telling me it was slowing down and it was heading back into my bad state.

I knew I had to get back on vitamin D3! And did. For the past eight months I have stuck to my daily intake of vitamin D3 at optimal doses.

When I think about these past eight months, something that sticks out to me is I am not as hungry. Because I am Italian, I eat a lot of pasta. Since I've been taking the vitamin D3, it's like it tells me when I need to eat and when I'm full and not to eat anymore. This is hard to explain, but it's like vitamin D3 got me to start listening to my body.

Now I simply shut down and don't feel like eating the wrong things or eating too much. It's like since I started taking ODA of vitamin D3 I have another layer of consciousness, now I listen to my body. It's very comforting, and my life has improved dramatically.

I sleep like a king, sleeping through the night. I very rarely wake up in the night. It's amazing.

I have not had a cold or the flu in almost three years.

I'm sharper at work and have more energy at work and with my family.

Today I'm at 187 pounds and I feel the best I have been in my life. Thank you, Dr. Somerville, and vitamin D3!

From Cathy Hoxworth in Laredo, Texas

I was a registered nurse living in McAllen, Texas, and my husband lived in Laredo. With all my nursing work and bending over so frequently, I often developed muscle knots in my back. A doctor in my hospital provided steroid shots whenever these pains flared up and became too painful.

After a number of shots, this doctor wanted to further investigate my pain problem, so he began a treatment of four shots over successive weeks. During the third shot, he punctured my somatic root nerve. That evening I started noticing a pain in my neck. The next morning my head was lying on my chest, and I was unable to move it up—not at all! I could not raise my head off my chest!

Nothing improved my status, and my head remained like this for one year.

About four months after this punctured nerve incident I started have burning sensations in my leg, and then in both my legs, and then in my right arm. This was very painful to the point where I could not touch them.

During this time, I worked with several doctors to find a solution and even traveled to Houston. Still, no doctor could find a way to improve my bent-forward head and all the pain in my limbs.

I was now wearing a neck brace and unable to perform my nursing duties. Because the doctors told me that nothing would cure this and since I could not work, I surrendered my nursing licenses after 1.5 years.

I had to move to Laredo so that my husband could take care of me.

After two years I went to visit Dr. Somerville who installed a morphine pump in both my hips and eventually another one in my neck for my arm pain. This helped ease the pain, but the downside of morphine is that it weakens your bones, which occurred. My bones were becoming brittle. Within two years I had broken my hip twice and had eleven of my teeth break off.

Dr. Somerville then diagnosed my condition as reflex sympathetic dystrophy (RSD) syndrome, a chronic disease that deteriorates the nerves, muscles, and bones; it is sometimes referred to as "chronic regional pain syndrome." There is no known cure, and it often it kills you because most people just give up.

And I was giving up. I was not able to get out of bed and get outside for five years! Being new to Laredo and now bedridden, I did not meet any people and had no friends in the area. All this was causing me severe depression. I still was scared to walk or go outside due to my brittle bones and pain. I was a mess and not feeling that I was getting better. I was worried and scared.

In response, Dr. Somerville switched my pump medication to fentanyl, which has improved my pain. Dr. Somerville also put me on vitamin D3 taking what he calls an "optimal dose."

Within two months I was shocked at my progress. I started sleeping through the night, which I hadn't done in five years. The pain in my legs and arms became manageable. I attribute this both to the new pain medication as well as vitamin D3 at optimal levels.

Now I am able to get out, make new friends, and be happy again. I was—and am—thrilled! I also got my appetite back because of my increased activity. I had gotten down to 79 pounds. Now I'm back up to 116 pounds.

By the way, I no longer wear my neck brace!

Vitamin D3 has changed my life. I still take the optimal dose of it every morning.

I know I would not be here today if it was not for Dr. Somerville. He saved my life! I love him very much.

From Laci Moffitt in Laredo, Texas

In May 2011, I turned 40 years old and got a "birthday" diagnosis of ovarian cancer... The next couple of years were filled with surgery, chemo, scans, and doctor appointments. My husband was friends with Dr. Somerville and would often talk to him about my situation for support and just to vent. Dr. Somerville mentioned to my husband that I should be taking vitamin D3, and that, in fact, everyone should be taking the miracle vitamin... I thought, "Well, it can't hurt," so I started taking it at Dr. Somerville's recommended optimal dose level.

My oncologist is amazed that I have not had a reoccurrence of ovarian cancer. He keeps telling me to keep doing whatever I'm doing. He says I'm a "miracle" because my type of ovarian cancer has a reoccurrence rate of 75% in the first couple of years. It's 2018—that's five years later—and I'm clean! Dr. Somerville has had something to do with it. I truly feel vitamin D3 is a part of my clean bill of health, and I tell everyone I know my story and to take vitamin D3 at optimal doses. Dr. Somerville and vitamin D3 saved my life.

From Brent Mainheart in Laredo, Texas

I have been a patient of Dr. Somerville for many years. I first went to see him after I had back surgery a number of years ago. After my back surgery I had an MRI, which showed that I had disc degeneration in both my back and shoulder.

In January 2011, I began taking optimal doses of vitamin D3 at the recommendation of Dr. Somerville. I was skeptical at first, but I took his word and wanted to try it. Within five weeks I started to notice a difference.

I recently went in to have another follow-up MRI done on my back and it showed that the degeneration had slowed down a lot! I attribute this to my vitamin D3 supplement routine.

Another benefit that has helped from taking vitamin D3 is that previously I had high cholesterol and now my levels are way down. I have not changed my exercise or my eating habits at all. So, the only thing I can attribute these positives things to is the intake of vitamin D3 supplements.

I have also noticed that my vision has improved, which has surprised everyone. In addition, my skin has improved.

I used to get sick with a cold or flu five to six times a year, but now I don't get sick at all.

I am getting the same number of hours of sleep, but I'm getting better sleep... more restful and peaceful sleep.

My wife has started taking vitamin D3 at optimal doses also. She has seen her skin improve and cholesterol levels lowered. She also has not had a cold since taking vitamin D3 where previously she had them frequently.

I give all the credit to Dr. Somerville and the vitamin D supplements that he recommended. He's given me my normal life back. Now I can pick up my seven-year old daughter and that means the world to me!

Glossary

clinical optimal blood level (COBL)—100–140 ng/ml—the blood levels that activate the maximum Madison-HannaH effects; the blood levels of vitamin D that allow deep restorative sleep, activate the summer metabolism, and fully boost the immune system, thereby essentially having your body work at its full potential and you in your healthiest state.

genotype—the gene or genes from a person's DNA that is responsible for a particular characteristic or trait.

gut—the part of the body that breaks down and absorbs food, in particular the stomach, small intestine, and large intestine.

gut flora—the bacteria, fungi and viruses among other living organisms that live inside the gut, particularly the large intestine.

Madison-HannaH effects—the effects that occur at COBL (see above); the effects of vitamin D that start only at much higher levels than currently recommended and that are necessary to fully turn on all the genes that boost a person's immune system, sleep, and metabolism to their most effective state.

optimal daily administration (ODA)—the daily dose of vitamin D3 that is typically required to obtain COBL (see above).

phenotype—the physical appearance of an organism based on the interaction of the organism's genes and the environment.

recommended dietary allowance (RDA)—the amount of a nutrient (or calories) considered necessary to maintain good health according to the Food and Nutrition Board of the National Research Council/National Academy of Sciences.

rickets—a disease that occurs in children resulting in a softening or weakening of bones. Typically it is due to an extreme and prolonged deficiency of vitamin D or rarely calcium or both.

telomere—a structure located on both ends of a chromosome; it is a region of repetitive nucleotides that ensures the integrity of a chromosome by preventing it from separating or fusing with other chromosomes.

vitamin D—the general term used to describe what is actually a secosteroid hormone. There are multiple different forms of vitamin D as the liver acts on it to produce the blood form, and the kidney acts to produce the active form in the blood. The active form that is produced in cells once the blood form reaches COBL is what activates the Madison-Hannah effects. There is also the form produced by mushrooms called vitamin D2. The form in fish and mammals is called vitamin D3.

vitamin D2—the form of vitamin D produced in mushrooms and often the main form of vitamin D used to supplement foods and liquids.

vitamin D3—the form of vitamin D that is produced by people's skin from sunlight exposure. It is also available as an over-the-counter supplement.

winter syndrome—the constellation or collection of diseases that occurs due to suboptimal blood levels of vitamin D. This syndrome results in sleep, immune system, and metabolism altering in anticipation of low sunlight levels, food scarcity, and the need to survive those periods. These changes are the ones that allow mammals typically to survive short periods of food scarcity, but when these changes are prolonged they cause winter syndrome due to the stress the changes put on the bodies. Winter syndrome can cause poor sleep, a weakened immune system, and obesity that then may result in diabetes, coronary artery disease, osteoporosis, and obesity, among others.

Acknowledgments

Thank you to Dr. Stasha Gominak, Dr. John Cannel, Dr. Mercola, and Dr. Scott. Thanks to Kathy Kazen for her countless hours editing my attempts to convey my thoughts. To David Line, Esq., for all the legal support and general counseling especially when things looked so, so, so bleak. To David Lizcano for his encouragement and support also during those dark times when all my friends were not to be found. To Jacques Simon, Esq., who was there when I needed him, trying to clean up a mess that others made, perhaps intentionally. To Maria Gonzalez and Rogelio De La O who were there throughout and supported me.

To the hundreds of my ex-patients who cared and encouraged me when I was in those dark days.

To my daughters who had to grow up fast but didn't flinch, and that made my life so much easier.

I would like to thank my editor Nancy Pile who made my words sing, kept me in line with addressing only one audience and without whom this book would never have been close to reaching its potential. Also, I thank Lise Cartwright for her coaching and recommending Nancy. Thanks to Kevin Ormsby for helping me develop a marketing plan to get my thoughts to others to read. He helped me more than he will ever know. Also, Alecia Ormsby for all her help in marketing and promoting my book. To those in the Self-Publishing School who encouraged me and helped me believe, both my fellow authors at Self -Publishing School who supported me and the experts there too—Sean Sumner, Eric Van Der Hope, and Chandler Bolt. To those at Bradley communications and the Quantum Leap program. Thank you to my fellow Quantum Leapers, Steve Harrison and all my indispensable coaches Martha Bullen, Geoffrey Berwind, Brian T. Edmondson, Debra Englander, Raia King and Rose George as well as Judy Cohen. I greatly appreciate my book designer Deana Riddle.

About the Author

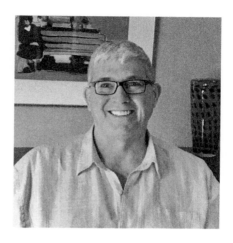

Judson Somerville, MD is a lifelong advocate for patients' health. His controversial approach to healthcare has been featured on the Today Show, MSNBC, in People Magazine, US News and World Report, and hundreds of newspapers around the world. He was also featured in a BBC special about his involvement in cloning the first human cells and advocating for those with chronic pain.

Dr. Somerville has practiced in the field of interventional pain management for more than two decades and has treated thousands of patients. He has authored or coauthored a dozen peer-reviewed articles and contributed a chapter on spine pain in a major textbook, *Practical Pain Management* (editors D.C. Tollison, J.R. Satterwhite, and J.W. Tollison).

Past president of the Texas Pain Society and the Small Districts Caucus of the Texas Medical Association, Dr. Somerville is constantly looking to improve his knowledge and the health of those under his care. When he became aware of the beneficial effects of vitamin D3, he researched the optimal dose and wrote this book to share his findings with readers looking for new solutions to their chronic health issues.

Visit Dr. Somerville's blog to learn more about the benefits of vitamin D3: www.vitamindblog.com.

Printed in Great Britain
by Amazon